HIJACKED BRAINS

HIJACKED

BRAINS

THE EXPERIENCE AND SCIENCE
OF CHRONIC ADDICTION

HENRIETTA ROBIN BARNES, MD

Dartmouth College Press | Hanover, New Hampshire

Dartmouth College Press
An imprint of University Press of New England
www.upne.com
© 2015 Trustees of Dartmouth College
All rights reserved
Manufactured in the United States of America
Designed by April Leidig
Typeset in Whitman and Scala Sans by
Copperline Book Services, Inc.

Figure 1.1 on page 28 is reprinted from *Current Opinion in
Neurobiology* 20, Leah H. Somerville and BJ Casey, "Developmental neurobiology of cognitive control and motivational
systems," 236–41, 2010, with permission from Elsevier.

Library of Congress Cataloging-in-Publication Data
Barnes, Henrietta N., author.
Hijacked brains: the experience and science of chronic
addiction / Henrietta Robin Barnes.
p. ; cm.
Includes bibliographical references and index.
ISBN 978-1-61168-674-6 (cloth : alk. paper)
ISBN 978-1-61168-675-3 (pbk. : alk. paper)
ISBN 978-1-61168-676-0 (ebook)
I. Title. [DNLM: 1. Chronic Disease — psychology. 2. Substance-
Related Disorders — psychology. 3. Behavior, Addictive —
psychology. 4. Drug Users — psychology. WM 270]
RC564.15
616.86 — dc23   2014018561

5 4 3

TO MY FAMILY
David
Jacob, Marsha, and Caleb
Rebecca and Shaun

CONTENTS

ACKNOWLEDGMENTS

I am most indebted to my patients with addiction or other chronic illnesses for sharing their stories and entrusting their health care to me. Russell Brazil and Jackie Smith-Darling first taught me what an addicted person's life can be like. Many others have enriched my understanding. To protect their anonymity, their names and details of their lives have been changed.

My mentors and colleagues have helped me become the person and doctor I am today. I gratefully carry their wisdom and interest with me. Nancy Leverich, a gifted high school English teacher, taught me how to write. Drs. LeClair Bissell, Ann Geller, and Leslie Davidson introduced me to the illness of addiction during medical school. In my internship at the Cambridge Hospital, Drs. Bill Clark, Margaret Bean-Bayog, and George Vaillant, each in his or her own way, modeled medical careers with addiction as a focus. In the early 1980s, the Commonwealth-Harvard Alcohol Research and Training (CHART) program, directed by Drs. Thomas Delbanco and Mark Aronson, put the primary care management of alcohol and other drug problems on the general internal medicine map. I am deeply grateful to them for including me in this project and to all my CHART colleagues, in particular Dr. JudyAnn Bigby and Donald Cutler, for this journey of discovery to a career in teaching, practicing, and writing about addiction in the primary care setting.

As interest in this field spread across the country and internationally, I had the opportunity to work with many people from different disciplines—family medicine, pediatrics, psychiatry, nursing, social work, and pharmacology. We were students, teachers, and mentors to each other. I would like to thank all of them for enriching my life. At the risk of omitting someone as I think back over the last thirty years of my career, I am particularly grateful to these people as colleagues and friends: Ted Parran, Jeffery Samet, Richard Saitz, John Knight, Peter Friedmann, Patrick O'Connor, Andy Spickard, Marianne Marcus, Mary-Ann Amodeo, Peggy Murray, Pat Kokotailo, Janet Williams, and Bud Isaacson.

Many of my colleagues and I stand on the shoulders of the small group of addiction specialists who founded the Association for Medical Education and Research in Substance Abuse (AMERSA). This organization has been my professional and academic home throughout my career. I am grateful to Dr. David Lewis and his cohorts, Drs. John Chappel, Sid Schnoll, Marc Galanter, and Eugene Schoener—among others—for their mentorship and pioneering efforts in addiction.

Writing this book has been a solitary process, but I am grateful for the assistance I received along the way. To clarify the science, several people explained their work to me. Special thanks to Mary Jeanne Kreek, Michelle Englund, Scott Swartzwelder, and Lucinda Miner and her colleagues at the National Institute on Drug Abuse. For policy and advocacy issues, David Rosenbloom was a gold mine of information.

I appreciate the input of Robert Bor, Pamela Thayer, Jacob Bor, Josefina Callender, Leslie Davidson, Richard Steinman, and Deborah Swiderski, who read early drafts of several chapters. Two people, David Bor and Robert Santulli, deserve my special gratitude for reviewing the entire manuscript and supporting me through the long gestation of this project.

The incisive comments of my editor, Phyllis Deutsch, helped me to hone the focus of this book. I am grateful for her insights, which have made this a much better story. For research, editorial, and artistic help at many points along the way, I would like to thank Alyssa Barrett, Malcolm Henoch, Peter Neill, Paul Bain, and Daniel Dugoff. I am particularly indebted to Sandy Trinh, my indefatigable research assistant, whose intelligence, hard work, computer savvy, and cheerfulness over the last several months have made this project a reality.

A special shout-out goes to my clinical colleagues and the staff at Cambridge Family Health for their patience and encouragement through the evolution of my primary care addictions practice and the many stages of this book project.

The love and support of my extended family and close friends have carried me through the ups and downs of writing my book. I particularly thank my husband, David Bor, for his wisdom, medical acumen, and sense of humor; my son, Jacob, for his thoughtful insights; and my daughter, Becca, for her empathy and ebullience. They and their families are the center of my life and precious to me beyond words.

The ideas and opinions in this book are mine alone, as is the responsibility for accuracy in content and references. I apologize in advance for any errors or omissions.

INTRODUCTION

Russell chose me as his doctor because, he told me, I didn't treat him "like an addict" when I first saw him for a drug-related problem. Over the next twenty years he showed me the possibility of living with grace, dignity, and addiction. At first glance, he had not appeared a likely candidate for that role. He was a stocky, muscular man. His rounded head with closely crew-cut hair merged imperceptibly into a thick, muscled neck. His eyes were hooded; his arms covered with tattoos and needle tracks; his teeth decayed and tobacco stained. He had the credentials to go with his menacing appearance: a childhood frayed by poverty and addicted parents, his own addictions, and a criminal record for drug dealing to support his addictions, his wife and son, and his lifestyle.[1]

However threatening he had been, the Russell I came to know was a gentle, caring man. He had struggled to get his addictions under control and had achieved complete remission from alcohol, heroin, and cocaine dependence. Nicotine was the toughest to give up. His rationale was that smoking was an addiction that harmed only himself. Knowing that stopping smoking was an absolute criterion for receiving the liver transplant he so badly needed, Russell still hesitated. He was not sure that he deserved to receive a transplant. His nicotine dependence and self-loathing conspired to delay a lifesaving surgical procedure. I do not know which he found more difficult: accepting a place on the transplant list or smoking his last cigarette.

He committed himself to a lifetime of treatment and support, which he found in the fellowship of Alcoholics Anonymous (AA), in our relationship, and most of all with his family. We celebrated his first, second, third, and fourth year of sobriety, and each successive one until he died sixteen years later of hepatitis C and liver cancer, complications of his alcohol and injection-drug use. He had spent twenty months on the two-year waiting list for a liver transplant.

As the hepatitis weakened him so that he could no longer work as a computer programmer, he worried constantly about providing for his wife and teenage son. As a dedicated member of his AA group, he sponsored countless other men trying to achieve remission from their addictions. I know the blessing of Russell's compassion. When my younger sister died in an accident, he comforted me at his next office visit, putting aside his own health issues. From early in my professional career, Russell taught me much of what I know about addiction. This was no intellectual exercise, but the lessons of a life redeemed.

Despite fifty years of evolving scientific understanding about addiction, prevalent sociocultural attitudes about addiction and people suffering with this disease are still embedded in beliefs and misconceptions common in the late nineteenth and early twentieth centuries. These attitudes have led and continue to lead to mistreatment of and discrimination against people with addiction. The goal of this book is to combat these misunderstandings with knowledge of the latest scientific research on addiction and the compassion and insight of a primary care physician who has cared for more than thirty years for people with chronic illnesses, including addiction.

Just a word about my work situation: My group practice is part of a public health care system in an ethnically and socioeconomically diverse city. On any day, the patients in our waiting room might include someone with chronic mental illness from a group home, a university professor with rheumatoid arthritis, an elected state official, an illiterate non-English-speaking woman with diabetes, a school principal with nicotine addiction, an unemployed laborer, and a lawyer with alcohol problems. Although addiction does not respect social or economic status, the precipitants and consequences of addiction mean that many of my addicted patients do live in poverty and depend on public health insurance. Addicted people with more resources and private health insurance often are better able to hide the ravages of addiction, but their desperation is the same. This book reflects my experience. Although at first glance my patients' stories may appear to reinforce common stereotypes, I urge the reader to keep in mind that over 90 percent of addicted people are indistinguishable from the rest of us.

Many Americans' lives are touched by addiction. One in four American families has a loved one suffering from addiction; family members struggle to understand this disease. Health care providers (nurses, psychologists, doctors, social workers), community safety personnel (police officers, firefighters), criminal justice workers, teachers, religious leaders, politicians, and policy makers—all need to understand addiction to do their work effectively. This book provides a basic understanding of addiction: what we know about it scientifically; how it is perceived and discriminated against in this country; and how it is lived by those suffering from it.

This book does not propose social or political solutions to our nation's drug problems. Nor will it provide advice for a family whose loved one has a drug problem. My intention is that those reading this book will recognize our country's deep social ambivalence about people with addiction and learn to treat the addicted person with compassion. An informed public will advocate for policies that address addiction as a chronic disease deserving of medical care and insurance, and neither marginalize nor stigmatize those with the condition.

My medical career has spanned a remarkable evolution in our understanding of addiction. We no longer consider alcoholism and drug dependence as distinct problems; they are both manifestations of addiction. We know that the course of addiction is much more complex than an inexorable downhill progression to death or to a miraculous recovery. We now understand that addiction is a chronic disease, like diabetes and heart disease, with periods of improvement and exacerbation. And as with many chronic illnesses, the most important treatment is learning to change to healthier behavior.

None of these thoughts were in my head as I walked into my first Alcoholics Anonymous meeting in the early 1970s, a required assignment from my medical school psychiatry professor. I did not want to be there. First, I had more important studying to do; second, I shared the disdain for alcoholics inculcated in me by more senior medical students, junior doctors, and senior faculty; and third, I felt self-conscious and alone among this group of middle-aged strangers. As the room quieted, the first speaker got up to tell his story of alcoholism. He launched into a horrific tale of drinking and more drinking, of blaming his wife for his drinking problems, of finding ways to drink on his job and getting fired, of being down and out, of stumbling into his first AA meeting intoxicated, of slowly returning to more meetings as his drinking lessened. Now he had been sober for a year; he was attending AA meetings several times weekly and learning to take his life "one day at a time." The audience greeted his story with laughter, applause, and gratitude for his sharing. I was astounded at the warmth and respect of the group for this person whom my colleagues might have called a "bum" or a "dirtball." And there I was, a socially responsible, diligent, but stressed medical student, feeling like an outsider. I could not fathom the sense of support and community among this group of normal, sober-looking folks who were apparently also all alcoholic. But I knew that I had seen something special and felt a tiny bit envious.

Despite the prevailing negative attitudes about alcoholism and drug addiction, which I now recognize as an expression of ignorance, not inhumanity, I continued to have unsettling epiphanies about these problems during my medical training. I learned that the overwhelming majority of my medical teachers knew a lot about the medical complications of alcoholism but almost nothing about the disease itself. A wonderful psychiatrist, whom I later learned was herself an alcoholic in recovery, taught me that my nascent empathy for people stigmatized because of their addiction was the essence of good doctoring, not the naivety of an inexperienced intern. When the head of a foundation, upset that a family member had received such poor treatment for alcoholism, offered one of my professors a grant to study alcohol problems in primary care medicine, I jumped at the chance to join the project. It turned out my professor did not know much about alcoholism in primary care; none of us did, not even the alcohol or drug specialists who cared mostly for patients with severe, progressive addiction in addiction treatment centers. We had to teach ourselves by sharing stories of our patients, talking with people in recovery, attending AA meetings, and trying to understand how someone who started as a social drinker could develop a problem as serious as alcoholism. We learned that addiction looks different in a primary care doctor's office, and requires a different approach, than addiction presenting as delirium tremens or end-stage liver disease, just as helping a patient in my office manage his high blood pressure and elevated cholesterol requires a different paradigm than the treatment of an acute heart attack in an intensive care unit. The idea that addiction was a prototypical primary care illness began to take form. Addiction has biological, psychological, and social dimensions; people suffering from addiction need ongoing medical care, whether their illness is in remission or they have relapsed. It is an illness that primary care providers can screen for, and that, if diagnosed and treated early, is likely to have better outcomes.

My passions as a primary care physician and an educator have been to take care of all my patients with chronic illnesses, including addiction, and to train others to care for and teach about people with addiction. The research and curiosity of my former students, colleagues, and many others have pushed forward our knowledge of addiction. My aim is to translate the evolution of our understanding of addiction over the last thirty years into a story that compels us to look at the science and to rethink how our society treats people with addiction.

My patients' lives are the heart of this book. Some have led coherent and productive lives with improvement in their addictions; others have doggedly pursued treatment after every relapse, in defiance of their progressive disease. And often their struggle has been a lonely one: they are spurned by family and friends they have betrayed, judged as deviant by the nurses and doctors who care for them, shunned by a society that perceives their behavior as selfish and immoral. This book follows the trajectory of people's struggles with addictive drugs, from their learning to use those drugs, to the science of brain dysfunction that may be triggered by use and lead to devastating consequences, and finally to addicted people's efforts to use whatever innate internal strengths and available external resources they have, or can learn, in order to get their illness into remission—to move from a state of overwhelming impulsive thoughts and behaviors to abstinence, toward learning how to work and to love again, or for the first time. Their courage humbles me; their lives are testaments to the durability of the human spirit.

If patients' stories are the heart of this book, clinical and social sciences form the backbone. The information I convey is based on up-to-date scientific research on genetics, neurobiology, brain development, as well as clinical and epidemiological studies. The field of clinical addiction is a relative newcomer to rigorous scientific investigation. New research technologies are increasing our understanding of addiction almost daily, but many of the researchers I spoke with cautioned me that we are far from putting all the pieces of the addiction puzzle together.

Chapter 1 elaborates how and why humans (and other species) learn to use addicting substances. Before developing addiction, our ancestors had to encounter mind-altering substances, either by finding them in nature or refining them through processes such as fermentation or, nowadays, synthesizing them in a laboratory. As a species we had to learn about these substances: How could they help us? What were the toxicities? What roles would societies assign to these substances? Human cultures have learned how to use addicting drugs positively (think of morphine for the relief of cancer pain) and negatively (the marketing of tobacco products despite knowledge of nicotine's addictive power and of tobacco's causal link to lung cancer). In essence, every adolescent or young adult recapitulates this history in learning to use a drug. Will I like alcohol? Will it make me sick? Will I want to use it again? As long as the benefits appear to outweigh the risks, the answer to the last question is likely to be yes. Underneath this simple linear process lies a web of explanations and questions that only gets more complicated as drug use progresses toward addiction. Studies on brain maturation, childhood developmental experience, family dynamics and traditions, peer pressure and social mores, genetics, and religion all contribute to our understanding of why teenagers are so vulnerable to initiating and continuing drug use.

An addicting substance or activity (gambling, sex) is a necessary, but not sufficient, component of addiction. Why can most people enjoy an addicting substance without problems while others develop addiction? Current neuroscientific research on addiction, the focus of chapter 2, provides insights into how deeply addiction affects basic brain activity. The survival of our species depends on neural circuitry that rewards us for sexual activity, staying well fed, and nurturing our children. There is nothing frivolous about these basic pleasures. Now imagine a substance that can hijack this reward pathway in the brain, so that a person's life revolves around anticipating, obtaining, and using this substance. Life's most essential activities are subsumed and governed by this powerful agent or activity to the detriment of everything else. This is addiction.

People struggle with addictions for many years. What is the natural course of this disease? Why do some get better, while others continue to deteriorate? In chapter 2, we turn to longitudinal studies with forty or fifty years of follow-up to learn that about one-third of addicted people improve, one-third get worse, and another third find a way to coexist with their addiction. However, for each individual, the course of addiction may be extremely variable. A person may move in and out of these categories of remission and relapse many times over a lifetime depending on her personal circumstances. Some addicted people with a positive outlook and good social skills demonstrate remarkable improvement; others are made more vulnerable by multiple losses, psychiatric illness, and economic circumstances.

As if addiction itself were not difficult enough, the stigma attached to it is pervasive. None of these addicted lives occurs in a cultural vacuum. Family attitudes, cultural customs, economic status, religious values, and government policies all affect how society regards addiction and how addicted people may feel about themselves. Chapter 3 chronicles just how complicated American attitudes about drug use and addiction have been since our country was founded and how this history has led to the stigma and discrimination that many addicted people face today. As a nation, we are ambivalent about any intoxicating substance used primarily for pleasure and enjoyment. The country was gripped by temperance fervor in the late nineteenth century, even as recent German immigrants were enjoying the social pleasures of their beer gardens. Today drinking alcohol is an accepted part of adult social activities for many people, while marijuana, a drug with similar short-term effects and a better safety profile, is reviled by many as a national scourge. The fact that one-third of the United States has decriminalized or legalized marijuana for medicinal or recreational reasons, while many other states still consider possession of small amounts of marijuana criminal behavior, indicates that we still disagree about the role of drugs in society. Our ambivalence applies not only to the drugs but to the communities that use them: contrast the fascination with cocaine use in glamorous Hollywood culture with the disapproval of crack cocaine use in inner-city African-American communities in the late twentieth century. We continue to be confused and ambivalent about addiction itself. Is it a brain disease with uncontrollable negative behaviors? A choice? A moral failing? A failure of willpower? A symptom of some other illness? A crime?

In chapter 3, we see that these persistent beliefs have real consequences for people with addiction. Stigma about addiction has led to discrimination in employment, housing, and education. The addiction treatment system is severely underfunded. Fewer than 15 percent of people with addiction ever access formal treatment, and treatment providers from physicians to counselors are overall poorly trained. Only 20 percent of the federal budget to address addiction issues goes to the health care system; 80 percent is used for criminal justice. What this chapter makes clear is that the "war on drugs" should not be an attack on the people who use drugs or have addiction.

The first three chapters examine the brain science of the disease of addiction and the social science of stigma and discrimination. The addicted person lives her life between these two forces. How does she negotiate between the distortions of an addicted mind and the hostile environment around her? What is it like to walk in her shoes? The next two chapters focus on patients' experiences of struggling with their addictions and the long, uneven process of recovery.

Chapter 4 discusses the interplay of genetic and environmental factors that determine one's vulnerability and resilience in the face of addiction. We discover that a person's response to addiction is multifactorial. During the process of human development, we are exposed to different kinds of risk at different ages. A newborn infant's dependence on the people in his environment makes him very vulnerable, just as the normal changes in an adolescent's developing brain increase the curiosity and impulsivity that may lead to very risky behaviors. Becoming addicted is itself a process with different rewards and risks as a person's disease progresses. And, of course, these changes occur in the complex reality of modern American life. A person's environments from the amniotic fluid of the womb, to a parent's capacity to nurture and care for a child, to peer pressure from schoolmates, to adult responsibilities of work and intimate relationships, pose intellectual, physical, and emotional challenges that can help someone manage his addiction or overwhelm and defeat him.

The slow process of recovery, of learning how to keep oneself safe from the allure of drugs, is the subject of chapter 5. Most people who develop addiction start drug use during adolescence, a critical period in maturation. Excessive use of drugs and addiction deprive an adolescent of experiences that would have helped him become independent, responsible, and capable of close, respectful relationships. It is not surprising that many people come to addiction treatment with the emotional maturity of a thirteen-year-old. Not only do they need to stop the addictive behavior; they need to function in a world that expects them to be adults, to assume roles and responsibilities for which they are often ill equipped. A solid recovery from addiction means not using drugs and also growing up, so that the addicted person has the maturity and skills to manage a relapse and live productively.

Before delving into the heart of the book, you will need some background information important to a basic understanding of addiction. In the remainder of this introduction, I will discuss and amplify the definition of addiction, and I want to convey what it is like to have a severe chronic illness. First, I shall discuss briefly some of the costs to society of addiction; then I will spend more time on the definition and chronic disease model of addiction.

The personal costs for people with addictions and their families are incalculable, but the social and economic burdens are well documented. The five leading causes of death in this country, which account for 70 percent of all adult deaths, are related to an underlying addiction—most commonly, to nicotine and alcohol.[2] Alone or in combination, these two drugs markedly increase the risk of heart disease, cancers of the mouth, throat, larynx, and lungs, stroke, and hypertension. The National Institute on Drug Abuse (NIDA) estimated that in 2008 the economic cost to society due to use of and addiction to tobacco, alcohol, and illicit drugs was $559 billion annually.[3] Addiction, like warfare, kills young adults just at the beginning of their productive work lives. In 2008, there were 36,450 deaths from drug overdoses, roughly equivalent to the total number of traffic accident fatalities that year.[4] In 2010, one-third of the 10,288 traffic fatalities due to alcohol-impaired driving occurred in the twenty-one to twenty-four-year-old age group.[5] Social scientists measure the impact of a disease on society in terms of the years of potential life lost if a person dies prematurely before the age of seventy or seventy-five. Between 2001 and 2005, the average annual deaths due to excessive alcohol consumption accounted for over 474,817 years of potential life lost (YPLL),[6] a magnitude comparable to YPLL in 2006 due to diabetes and stroke combined. Violence, prostitution, fatal overdoses, and life-threatening infections take their toll on injection-drug users, their families, and both the health care and criminal justice systems.

On a much brighter note, a 2008 report on data collected and analyzed over the previous fifteen years indicates that effective substance abuse (SA) prevention programs for communities and schools do exist. If effective school-based SA prevention programs were implemented nationally, the annual savings would be about $100 billion, or a savings of eighteen dollars for each student.[7] Unfortunately, over 80 percent of students receive either no SA education or programs of no or marginal effectiveness, which includes the ubiquitous D.A.R.E. (Drug Abuse Resistance Education) program.[8] Prevention may ultimately be the most important tool in reducing the burdens of addiction. What is this illness that is so destructive to our society?

The essence of addiction is the compulsive use of a substance or other behavior despite known negative consequences. The World Health Organization (WHO) defines addiction in terms of substance dependence: "A cluster of behavioral, cognitive, and physiological phenomena that develop after repeated substance use and that typically include a strong desire to take the drug, difficulties in controlling its use, persisting in its use despite harmful consequences, a higher priority given to drug use than to other activities and obligations, increased tolerance, and sometimes a physical withdrawal state."[9]

Let's take this definition apart. First, it describes a pattern of behavior over time. A complex combination of forces compels the activity. Sometimes it is the force of habit. How many of us have taken one of several familiar routes to work and arrived unable, momentarily, to remember which route we took? We were on automatic pilot—our bodies and brains were performing complicated activities while some of our attention was elsewhere. So too with addiction. Changes in the brain may trigger complicated drug-seeking behaviors, even as my patient professes a desire not to drink. Just last week, a young man trying to stay off opioids told me, "I don't want to use—even when I find myself using, I don't want to use." Is my patient simply lying, telling me what he thinks I want to hear, as some of my colleagues would allege? Or, as I have come to understand, is this contradiction a fundamental aspect of addiction dictated by changes in the addicted brain? I cannot fault my colleagues for their opinions. Inadequate medical education about addiction has left many physicians ill prepared for caring for addicted patients.[10] Ignorance is a fertile field for myths and stereotypes.

Sometimes the compulsion to use drugs is fueled by a need to escape intolerable pain, unbearable reality, or just to feel "normal." JL, a woman in her late thirties now on stable methadone maintenance treatment, describes her predicament in a documentary film about opiate addiction and recovery.[11] At the start of her heroin use, she was a single mother with five children. The year before, both her father and her husband had died. She was in a body cast for injuries suffered in a car crash. She felt overwhelmed by responsibility, grief, poverty, and pain.

"It was just too much," she says. Heroin offered at least temporary relief. When she tried heroin, she reports, "I felt like I had no problems. I felt like I was walking on clouds."

Her situation was extreme, but the normal unpleasant emotions—anger, rejection, loss, loneliness, sadness, frustration, hopelessness—that most people find ways to tolerate or get through feel unbearable for the addicted person and fuel drug use.

Substance use. Caffeine or coca, alcohol or heroin, nicotine or prescription painkillers, cocaine or marijuana—each drug acts on various brain receptors and, through a series of mechanisms, ultimately affects the brain's reward pathway. Over time, repeated drug use carves a path in the brain's landscape. This pathway is no pretty garden walk but a well-traveled and familiar trail, ultimately not to the brightness of pleasure but to darkness and pain.

Other addictive behavior. Certain activities, such as compulsive gambling, can also trigger these neural pathways. In fact, even the anticipation and arrangement of such activities can provide pleasure more intense than the pleasure of the activity itself. The positive memories formed around those activities play a critical role in maintaining the behavior. Just think how anticipation about that trip to a favorite resort in Florida next March helps you get through the dark days of December and January.

Known negative consequences. Unfortunately, the adverse consequences of addiction can affect every aspect of life: personal health, self-esteem, family relationships, social activities, financial status, ability to work, and exposure to legal sanctions—whether driving under the influence of alcohol or purchasing an illicit drug. This brief list belies the devastation of addiction. While people with addictions may publicly deny or minimize the consequences of their behavior, they all live with a painful awareness of its destructive consequences, even as they see drugs as the immediate solution to their problems.

You may have noted that I keep referring to addiction and not to alcoholism or heroin dependence or cocaine abuse or compulsive gambling as separate entities. Addiction describes the common underlying compulsion. What *drug* addiction looks like, as a specific example, depends on the pharmacological effects of the drug and its legal or illegal status. American society permits the use of caffeine, nicotine, and alcohol for pleasure. Most other drugs are proscribed; distribution and trafficking are harshly punished. On the other hand, coca is acceptable in Bolivia, and several states have decriminalized the use of marijuana for medical or legal reasons, despite federal laws prohibiting it. The illegal status of many addictive drugs and the criminal behavior of some drug users (driving while intoxicated, stealing, and violence) obscure the fact that the underlying problem is a chronic, treatable disease.

Addiction is a chronic illness, and chronic illnesses have no cure. Their course, measured in years, is marked with periods of relapse and remission. As with diabetes, hypertension, or arthritis, there are medications to treat the condition, but the most important treatment is learning new adaptive behaviors.

When EM recently walked into my office with a big smile on her face, I hardly recognized her. She radiated energy and pride. The EM I remembered from the previous year had problems taking care of herself; her visits to my office were sporadic; overweight, she did not follow any specific diet or take her medication regularly. Providing for her young children had taken priority over managing her chronic illness. Now, EM told me, she had gone on her own to a special clinic for her illness. The clinic's strict program had helped her turn the corner. She lost over twenty pounds, began to exercise regularly, and educated herself about her illness. The specialist had made only minor changes in her medications, but her illness—diabetes—was now well controlled. She will always have diabetes, but she has taken charge. She wants to prevent the most serious consequences of diabetes—heart disease, kidney failure, blindness—from interfering with her life. And yet, her recent blood test results tell me that keeping her diabetes in good control will always be a struggle.

DC has had to work harder to manage her illness. She had tried to make the necessary changes in her life but kept slipping back to old behaviors. When she did manage to get her illness into remission, she continued to need treatment three to four times weekly. When I first met her, she had recently married and moved into a new home. She was managing a busy dental practice. Her life seemed so together and, well, normal, that her insecurity about her illness appeared unwarranted. As I have learned over time, DC knows her illness better than I do. Another severe relapse could destroy everything that she has worked so hard to achieve. She continues in treatment three times a week, because, as she explained, "my life depends on it." DC has cocaine addiction, in remission for more than twenty years.

As young women, neither of these patients thought that her illness could disrupt her life and health. A lifetime of managing a long-term illness was not what either had bargained for. There is no cure around the corner for them to look forward to, just the vigilance of keeping the illness under control day after day after day. And even so, EM's blood sugar levels can spiral out of control, or DC's craving for cocaine may overwhelm her. Should either one relapse, she will need more intensive treatment to get her illness under control again and to understand what triggered these old, unhealthy patterns. This knowledge will help her prevent future relapses.

Chronic illnesses have different causes and varied courses. They require different medications, and the details of management are unique for each illness and each individual. My patients with osteoarthritis in their knees and hips need to lose weight and stay active despite the pain. People with high blood pressure have a disease initially without symptoms, yet they need to juggle medications with annoying side effects. My addicted patients need to avoid their drug of choice and possibly take medication to decrease the likelihood of using their drug, while they slowly learn the cognitive and emotional skills needed to repair their damaged lives and keep themselves safe from relapse. No pill alone will take care of a chronic illness. All these illnesses require significant changes in behavior. The determination of people like EM and DC to engage daily in a struggle that never ends and, despite their best efforts, may eventually defeat them inspires my respect and admiration.

One can understand the impact of any chronic illness only by trying to see the world through that person's eyes. Many of my patients cope with a chronic illness while juggling family responsibilities, a job, and the demands of their illness. For other patients, managing their illnesses is a full-time job.

SB developed type 1 diabetes at age fourteen. He had to learn to eat a diabetic diet, test his blood sugar levels, and inject insulin twice a day. Thirty years later, he sits in my office, his thin body clad in blue jeans and a T-shirt. The swollen tips of his fingers look like ten tiny pincushions from testing his blood sugar at least eight times a day. To manage his diabetes and care for his young son, he has had to give up his job as a videographer. Despite meticulous attention to his diabetes, he now has devastating complications of diabetic neuropathy. His digestive system cannot move food along normally, so that even a small meal causes fullness and bloating. His bladder no longer works independently, so that he has to use a catheter. Worst of all, he has incapacitating nerve pain in his legs and hands that is marginally controlled with multiple medications. SB is not a complainer, but he sums up the fatigue of dealing with his diabetes and of living with excruciating pain this way: "It's always with you; there is never a day off."

DK would agree. At eighty-four, she takes twelve medications to stabilize her heart failure, emphysema, arthritis, hypertension, and glaucoma, to name only the most active illnesses. With any exertion—think dressing, think bathing—she feels breathless and may have chest pain. Her knees are too painful for walking. Her mobility is a wheelchair, limiting her world to her tiny apartment. Yet, she perseveres, sometimes with grim determination, often with an acerbic wit, describing a recent fall as if she were a dancer practicing a difficult step.

In my work as a general internist in the community, I cure very few illnesses. The colds and backaches will resolve within weeks no matter what I do. Antibiotics will cure some infections, or pain medicine will help someone through an acute injury. Sophisticated medical technology such as DK's pacemaker or SB's insulin pump has made many illnesses more manageable. While new medications and modern science may have slowed the decline, the nature of most chronic illnesses is gradual progression.

Imagine managing multiple medications daily, scheduling therapies and physician visits and perhaps transportation as well, learning to pace yourself to avoid exhaustion, trying to maintain relationships with family and friends, struggling to pay your bills because you cannot work the way you used to, giving up foods or habits that once brought pleasure or comfort. And the best you can hope for is that things won't get worse too quickly. From a distance, the picture is grim. Up close, there's the triumph for SB of learning to let go of things he cannot change; for DK, the joy of a walk outside, wheeled by her daughter-in-law. For Russell, there was the quiet acceptance that his hard-won sobriety would not free him from the ravages of his illness.

As with diabetes or osteoarthritis, a majority of people with addictions manage the ups and downs of their illness without requiring hospitalization. They need to find a way to live with their disease that decreases the harm to themselves and others and lets them live as full a life as possible. But the ravages of their particular illness may limit their options. Just as we would not expect someone with advanced multiple sclerosis to get up and walk or a woman with metastatic ovarian cancer to stay in remission forever, people with severe addiction may be able to forestall the damage of their disease, but they too may succumb to it.

Chronic illness usually develops gradually and may be relatively asymptomatic for years. By the time breast cancer is suspected from an abnormal mammogram or physical examination, the cancer has been present for at least four or five years. Often early diagnosis and intervention can either prevent or decrease the effects of a chronic disease. Simple screening tests such as checking a person's blood pressure or performing a Pap smear help to prevent heart disease or cervical cancer, a common cancer in women. Once highly active antiretroviral therapy was available to control the progression of HIV/AIDS, the numbers of people requesting screening skyrocketed. Substance misuse, whether part of addiction or not, has many of the characteristics of the above diseases. It is common, develops over years, and effective treatment can decrease the morbidity and mortality. Fortunately, there are effective screening techniques and effective early interventions that can help a person change his use of a particular substance. And for those with more severe addiction, behavioral therapies and new medications have shown very promising results.

Use of drugs may be risky depending on the drug, the person, and the circumstances. Clearly, a combination of heavy drug use, personal vulnerabilities, and environmental pressures is likely to result in unfortunate outcomes. However, most people can enjoy alcohol or caffeine in moderation without endangering their health. There are some people who use opiates or cocaine for enjoyment and without health problems, but the potential risks are higher.

On the other hand, established addiction is neither a pleasure nor a choice. Any illness that deprives a person of his ability to perceive reality, to make reasonable decisions, to feel in control of his own life, and to have hope for the future is a heavy burden indeed.

My goal is to have the reader understand addiction from both the scientific and the human perspective. The purpose is to weave together these two threads—one of statistical data and scientific evidence; the other from clinical data of patient care, data from the human heart that is the essence of medical care. As Francis Weld Peabody, a well-known Boston physician in the early twentieth century, noted, "The secret of the care of the patient is in caring for the patient."[12]

This book follows the stories of five of my patients. All the events recorded did occur, but names and details have been changed to protect anonymity. Several other patients, identified by their initials, make cameo appearances. After the deaths of Jackie Smith-Darling and Russell Brazil, their respective spouses gave permission for me to use their names and stories. I am grateful to Russell and Jackie for sharing their lives with me and to their spouses for allowing me to share their resilience and courage in the face of addiction.

I would like to introduce here the five main "characters" as I first met them, so that the reader can follow their lives more easily:

Delia is a twenty-six-year-old woman from a suburban family who began using drugs after her first year of college. She worked as a bartender and waitress, but a violent relationship led to frequent relapses. When she decided to get sober, she threw out her cell phone with all her drug connections. She struggles with depression, attention deficit disorder, and post-traumatic stress disorder (PTSD.)

Linda is a thirty-three-year-old single mother, ambivalent about separating from her addicted husband who had introduced her to drugs at age fifteen. Her two daughters are finishing elementary school; she has just landed a two-month seasonal job at Toys "R" Us. She suffers from bipolar disorder and PTSD from two years living on the street doing drugs, while her aunt and uncle took care of her daughters.

Bill, a thirty-two-year-old heavy drinker who switched to injecting heroin after his younger brother died ten years ago, has worked as a laborer and on construction. He has been unemployed for several years and lives with his mother. He is frustrated and angry and feels the whole world is against him.

Larry, now twenty years old, lost his mother in a car crash when he was fifteen. Estranged from his father, his life fell apart. He dropped out of school, started using heroin when he could no longer afford prescription painkillers, and was on probation for a drug-related offense. Referred to me by a detoxification center, he has been off heroin for just five days.

Martha is a fifty-two-year-old widow estranged from the only family she has, a twenty-five-year-old addicted son. She has been through multiple detoxifications from alcohol and clonazepam (Klonopin). Just discharged from a month-long residential program, she is hopeful and confident that she can stay sober.

This book explores my patients' and others' experiences of drug use and addiction. Scientists have explained their complicated research to me. Other physicians have told me about their patients. People with addiction have trusted me with their stories. At the end of each interview, I have asked, "What do you think is most important for the American public to understand about addiction?" This book is my attempt to do justice to their answers.

ONE

LEARNING TO USE

It smells sweet and spicy, and I drink deeply before I realize what a terrible first drink it is. On my tongue, the flavor is completely foreign, a revolting combination of black licorice and antiseptic. I swallow it like a carnival freak swallows fire and can feel its red glow in my throat.—Koren Zailckas, *Smashed*

So Koren Zailckas describes her first alcoholic drink in her autobiography, *Smashed: Story of a Drunken Girlhood.*[1] Over the next few pages, she relates how she learned to drink alcohol: how she got beyond the unpleasant taste, how she began to anticipate its positive effect of relieving her shyness. She learned that if one drink is good, two or three or four would be better. Like many people learning to drink, she also drank too much. At age sixteen, she had already had one Emergency Department visit for acute alcohol poisoning.[2] Unlike most people, she did not learn to modify her drinking to maximize the benefits and minimize the hangovers, embarrassing episodes, and associated risky behaviors. That calculus of the risks and benefits of using drugs is different for each individual and changes as people mature and take on more adult roles. Most people are able to find a balance that allows them to enjoy their drug of choice in moderate amounts without harmful effects. Not Koren, whose attempts to cope with desperate unhappiness led to alcohol abuse and eventual recovery. . . . Why is using drugs a behavior that so many people want to learn?

The Universality of Drug Use

Human beings have used substances to create altered states of consciousness for eons. Evidence of early human use of opium has been found in Neolithic lakeshore dwellings in Switzerland.[3] The poppy played an important role in cultures of the Middle East, most probably starting in Mesopotamia and spreading west to Egypt and to Greece.[4] According to mythology, Demeter, the Greek earth goddess, carried a sheaf of poppy flowers as she searched for her lost daughter, Persephone. Hippocrates, a physician in ancient Greece, is said to have been intrigued with the powers of opium as a soporific and pain reliever, but warned of its addicting effect on the brain. Over the next two thousand years, cultures in Asia and Europe ascribed various medicinal powers to opium, but not until the advent of tobacco and smoking in the late 1600s did opium prepared for smoking (*chandu*) enjoy widespread popularity as a recreational drug used by wealthy people in East Asia.[5] Interestingly, the epidemic of opium smoking among Chinese in the eighteenth and nineteenth centuries was fueled by the aggressive trading tactics of the British East India Company.[6] Over the protestations of successive Chinese leaders, the transport of opium from the Indian subcontinent to the vast potential markets of China was too lucrative for the British to give up.

Other drugs played a central role in different cultures. Bacchus, the god of wine, attested to the importance of alcohol in ancient Greco-Roman culture. In the Western Hemisphere, hallucinogens played a major role in tribal cultures. Indigenous North Americans used high doses of tobacco.[7] Shamans in the northwest Amazon region believed hallucinogens could turn them into jaguars and give them power to contact and to some degree manipulate the spirit worlds.[8] Until alcohol was introduced to the Eskimo people by the British and French in the eighteenth century, they were the only known ethnic and cultural group in the world not using some mind-altering drug.[9]

Humans are not the only animals to use mind-altering substances. As Michael Pollan points out in *The Botany of Desire,* a wonderful treatise on the relationship between plants and animals, a plant may produce a chemical as a defense against its predators, sometimes with unexpected consequences. Some of these plant chemicals activate the reward system in the animal's brain, so that the animal returns again and again to the plant until its intoxicated brain can no longer function. He mentions locoweed for cattle and hallucinogenic lichens for grazing sheep, but saves his descriptive genius for his cat's reaction to catnip:

> Every summer evening at around five, Frank would lumber into the vegetable garden for a happy hour nip of *Neptaria cataria,* or catnip. He would first sniff, then tug at the leaves with his teeth and proceed to roll around in paroxysms of what looked to me like sexual ecstasy. His pupils would shrink to pinpricks and take on a slightly scary thousand mile stare, preparatory to pouncing on unseen enemies or—who can say—lovers. Frank would crash-land in the dirt, pick himself up, do a funny little sidestep, then pounce again until, exhausted, he'd go sleep it off in the shade of a tomato plant.[10]

The persistence of such drug-using activity over time, geography, and species suggests that using psychoactive substances fills a compelling need or desire in human and animal brains. However, only humans have found ways to alter these drugs in both agricultural and manufacturing stages. Belladonna, known familiarly as deadly nightshade for its toxic properties, has given us atropine, a medication used in surgery and in heart disease. Morphine, derived from opium, remains one of the most effective medicines we have to relieve the suffering of severe pain. Hallucinogens, including lysergic acid diethylamide (LSD), were once used to help people in psychotherapy expand their consciousness. On the dark side, we have taken the coca leaf, a mild stimulant when used in tea or chewed, and converted it into the devastatingly addictive drug cocaine.

Drug use may be a near-universal human experience, but societies have different and complex relationships with the drugs used by their members. We can divide use of psychoactive substances into four broad categories:

1. Spiritual or ritual activities.
2. Relief of pain in its many forms.
3. Aids to help us cope with daily life.
4. Pleasure: happiness, relaxation, increased sense of power or sexuality, mind "expansion" for intellectual or emotional curiosity. The pleasures of using drugs are as varied as the people who use them.

Many cultures employ drugs as part of religious rituals. The most familiar to many American readers may well be the Christian Eucharist, the sacred ritual performed by Jesus on the first night of Passover before his arrest and crucifixion: "And he took a cup, and when he had given thanks he gave it to them saying, 'Drink of it, all of you; for this is my blood of the covenant, which is poured out for many for the forgiveness of sins'" Matthew 26:27–28.[11] For more than two millennia, the Jewish people have maintained this ritual of celebrating the Passover seder with wine. In contrast, other religions or fundamentalist sects forbid any use of alcohol. This absolutism obviates the need to grapple with a behavior that can cause both pleasure and harm. For Muslims, the Qur'an describes drinking as an abomination in this life but promises rivers of wine in the afterlife.[12]

Pain may well be the most universal human experience, and its forms affect us in different ways: physical pain from an injury or surgery, emotional pain from loss or psychological trauma, the discomfort and danger of withdrawal from addictive drugs. It is not surprising that relieving pain is a human preoccupation. Our own brains produce chemicals that can aggravate or calm reactions to pain. The most potent pain medicines are opioids, including opiates derived from the opium poppy (opium, morphine, heroin, codeine) and the synthetic opioids (hydrocodone [Vicodin], oxycodone [Percocet], methadone, and others). All these drugs mimic our own natural painkillers, endorphins, but with much stronger effect. The opioids, along with alcohol and other sedatives (barbiturates, benzodiazepines such as diazepam [Valium] or alprazolam [Xanax]) also blunt our perception of pain. Sir William Osler, arguably the most well-known American physician of the nineteenth century, paid homage to opium by referring to it as "God's own medicine."[13] When I ask heroin-addicted women what they like most about heroin, the usual answer is, "It makes me numb. I don't have to feel anything." These women struggle not only with addiction but also with loss of family members to drugs and violence, and a profound sense of worthlessness and hopelessness. Marijuana affects the brain's endocannabinoid receptors (CB1 receptors), which modulate a myriad of neural interactions involved with perception, emotion, and the effects of other drugs. Alcohol may also serve this numbing function, as Koren Zailckas learned only too well.[14] Finally, anyone whose body is used to large doses of pain medicines—whether a patient with cancer pain or one addicted to heroin—will have severe discomfort if the medicine is stopped abruptly. Restarting the drug will eliminate these withdrawal symptoms promptly.

Sometimes just getting through the day seems tough enough, even without a particular pain problem. Caffeine and nicotine, both stimulants, are the most common drugs in the American workplace today. In the mid-nineteenth century, small amounts of opium made working conditions more tolerable for the Chinese immigrants toiling in mines and building the transcontinental railroad.[15] Today, as they have for centuries, Bolivian miners chew coca leaves as a mild stimulant to ward off hunger and enhance their ability to sustain physical work[16] at the Andes' high altitudes.

The use of drugs solely for pleasure taps a nerve of ambivalence that runs deep in American society. We condone drinking alcohol, especially in the context of a meal or a particular celebration. However, drinking to out-of-control intoxication, the normative pattern for many adolescents and young adults, is definitely not acceptable to mature older adults because of the risky behaviors associated with intoxication. Smoking tobacco shared the same acceptance as alcohol until the publication in 1968 of the *Surgeon General's Report on Smoking*, which linked tobacco with heart and lung diseases and confirmed smoking as a cause of lung cancer.[17]

In the second half of the twentieth century, artists, intellectuals, and entertainers (in the vanguard or at the margin of American culture, depending on your perspective) popularized several of today's illicit drugs. The early 1950s saw Beat-generation writers such as Allen Ginsberg, William Burroughs, and Jack Kerouac explore marijuana use as an aid for artistic creativity. For Ginsberg, smoking marijuana was also a moral declaration of his First Amendment rights and a protest against what he experienced as the stifling and repressive culture of the McCarthy era. The use of hallucinogens, particularly LSD, followed marijuana as an expression of freedom and creativity. As Timothy Leary put it in a conversation with the author Martin Torgoff, "Our precise surgical target [in using these drugs] was the Judeo-Christian power monolith, which had imposed a guilty, inhibited, grim, anti-body, anti-life repression on

Western civilization."[18] In looking back on his experience with psychedelic drugs, Peter (Cohon) Coyote, a member of the San Francisco Mime Troupe, echoed, "Psychedelics did to our perceptions of reality what Einstein did to Newtonian physics."[19] LSD users envisioned themselves heralding a new era of relative reality that would return America to its ideals of personal freedom and liberty.

The conflicting experiences of the American drug scene bring us back, time and again, to long-unsettled, and unsettling, questions: At what point should public health and safety take precedence over individual choice or industry profits? Conversely, if most people can enjoy a drug without experiencing problems, is harm to a few sufficient cause to ban its use? At what point should society curtail the "pursuit of happiness" of most citizens in order to promote the public health and safety of a small minority who use a drug irresponsibly or develop addiction?

Adolescence: The Age of Initiation to Drug Use

Larry, Delia, and Linda all started using drugs as adolescents, as most people do. Several national studies over the last twenty years have documented the initiation of drug use in teenage years.[20] Throughout that time period, about one-half of drug initiates have been adolescents under eighteen.[21] This pattern has remained constant even though the total number of adolescents starting to use drugs has varied. From a nadir in the early 1990s following the Reagan administration, initiation of drug use has increased steadily until leveling off in the last several years. The annual Monitoring the Future study, funded by the National Institute on Drug Abuse, has documented that between 1991 and 2012 the lifetime prevalence of substance use among high school seniors decreased for alcohol (from 88 to 70 percent) and cigarettes (from 63 to 40 percent) and increased for marijuana (from 36 to 45 percent).[22] This pattern of drug initiation in adolescence is similar in Canada, Mexico, Brazil, Germany, and the Netherlands, whereas the prevalence (absolute number) of users of alcohol, cannabis, and opiates varies widely among these countries.[23]

Social norms and family customs play a significant role in a child's initiation of drug use.[24] Caffeine in the form of colas and other soft drinks is the most common psychoactive drug used by children. Caffeine is consumed by 87 percent of Americans over the age of two,[25] and caffeine addiction is sanctioned by our society. All other drugs, with the exception of those prescribed for medical conditions, are illegal for American children to use until the age of eighteen for tobacco products and the age of twenty-one for alcohol.[26] Nevertheless, parents are potent role models for children's behaviors. Children of parents who smoke cigarettes are twice as likely to smoke cigarettes as the children of nonsmokers, despite verbal messages about the dangers of smoking.[27] Alcohol is a different story. Cultural traditions and health messages that one to two drinks of alcohol daily may be beneficial give alcohol a more accepted role in the home.[28] Some families, especially those of southern European and Mediterranean heritage, drink wine as a beverage at meals and may introduce their children to wine at a young age. Children will absorb their families' attitudes and practices of alcohol use, whether or not they are specifically taught to drink at home. The United States and the United Kingdom are the only developed countries that regulate children's drinking age at home. Children whose families and friends do not drink alcohol are unlikely to encounter alcohol until adolescence. If their adolescent peers do not drink, abstinent behavior is reinforced. But if their adolescent peers do drink, the forbidden nature of alcohol may increase its allure.

While parents everywhere worry about the possible consequences of their teens' experimentation with drugs, we need to recognize that exploring the environment and taking risks is normative behavior for a teenager. Most teenage users are experimenters with drugs, not individuals with substance use disorders. Developmental psychologists tell us that adolescent children are learning to be independent of their parents. Teens dress differently, may use different language, and appear to reject (at least temporarily) family values. They may assert their independence with risky behaviors that often involve experimenting with substances. Adolescents' inability to take account of the future consequences of their actions promotes a sense of invulnerability. Their impulsiveness may overcome their emerging better judgment. A recent study using data from the *Development of the Person*[29] demonstrated that teen experimentation with alcohol and marijuana at seventeen-and-a-half predicted better adjustment at age twenty-six in four domains: more education compared with abstainers, a better work ethic than those with drug abuse or dependence as teens, and more involvement with romantic relationships and better overall functioning than the "at risk" users.[30]

The Developing Brain

New research in neurobiology and social science has added a dimension of scientific evidence to previously theoretical discussions about adolescent behavior. A look at normal brain development will help us understand whether and how initiating drugs may be problematic for the adolescent brain. Some of the neurobiological research is based on imaging techniques developed in the last two decades.[31] These techniques allow researchers to take detailed pictures of the structure and the function of the brain and compare them over time.[32] We know that a person's brain continues to develop and change throughout the life span, reaching maturity by the mid- to late twenties. This maturation reflects both progressive and regressive changes in different areas of the brain as it responds to genetic and environmental stimuli. Scientists have coined the term "plasticity" to describe the brain's ability to change patterns of growth and connectivity. Any brief, simplified description of the brain's function belies its elegant complexity but may help orient the reader to the basic vocabulary of neuroscience. Early writers, unable to determine functional areas of the brain, simply described the brain as made up of "gray matter" and "white matter." Gray matter consists of billions of neural cells. These cells can accept, hold, and move molecule-size bits of information. They accept sensory input (taste, pain, fear, beauty) and send a signal for a response (pucker, cry out, run, smile). Some bits of information are useful, even crucial, to functioning; many other bits are irrelevant or confusing. Think how difficult it can be to carry on a conversation at a crowded party, while your brain is busy screening out other voices and loud music. The brain must be able to suppress extraneous information all the time. In order to be effective, brain cells require an organizational structure and a way to communicate with each other. This is where the white matter comes in, providing the connectivity—the wires, if you will—between areas of gray matter that need to communicate (e.g., touch hot stove > pain > remove finger > scream > put finger in ice water). Over time, white-matter cells develop a myelin sheath that improves their conductivity. At the same time, there is trimming of the dendrites, branches of the neural cells, in the gray matter to eliminate excess or confusing signaling. As the brain matures, organization and connectivity develop, while the "disconnected" gray matter is pruned.[33] These changes are triggered by activation of genes deep within cell nuclei in response to messages from inside and outside the cell. Environmental experiences like severe traumatic stress or the repetitive use of addicting drugs can alter or override the normal development of communication pathways between brain cells.

Let's look at what the science of normal children's brains tells us. Magnetic resonance imaging (MRI) shows that the sequence of the maturation process in the human brain parallels the observable childhood developmental milestones.[34] The parts of the brain controlling sensation and movement mature first, followed by temporal and parietal areas, which govern basic communication skills. Cognitive abilities appear to develop in a linear manner from childhood to adulthood. In childhood, the signaling from the limbic (emotional) system and the prefrontal cortex, or PFC (cognitive), are in relative balance. Adolescence brings a surge in emotionality and reward seeking that can overpower a teen's cognitive abilities.[35] The ability to modulate feelings, perform complex cognitive tasks, delay gratification, and inhibit inappropriate behaviors is driven by the development of the prefrontal cortex in late adolescence and early adulthood (fig. 1.1). As the connecting nerve cells develop, the higher-function areas of the brain exert a "top down" ordering and control of the emotional and reward-related impulses initiated by the midbrain.[36] These neurobiological changes during adolescence explain the gradual development of abstract thought, judgment, and impulse control.

Adolescence, from puberty to the emergence of an independent, autonomous adult, is a turbulent time for brain development. Pubertal hormones and opportunities for novel experiences stimulate the limbic areas of the brain involved in emotions, motivation, and reward. Teens have an exaggerated limbic reaction and increased physiologic response to emotional cues, positive or negative, with diminished cognitive control. The end of a brief romance can make a teen feel that life is not worth living. The allure of hanging out with friends after school may trump the responsibility of studying for tomorrow's physics exam. Alter-

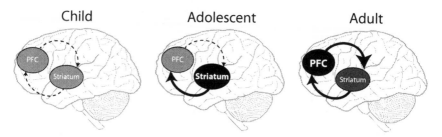

Fig. 1.1 Model of striatal (needs, wants) and prefrontal cortical (cognitive controls) functional interconnections across development. Dotted arrows represent immature connections; solid arrows represent mature connections.

natively, the anticipated approval from parents and teachers for a good grade may send the student to the library. While parents might prefer the goal-directed behavior of the studious teen, it is important to realize that, in both these scenarios, the driving force is the salience of the emotional reward rather than a rational assessment of future consequences. This imbalance between emotional reward seeking and cognitive control makes adolescence a particularly vulnerable time to be experimenting with drugs and alcohol.[37]

Do Adolescent and Adult Brains Respond Differently to Drugs?

We need to know whether drugs act differently in the brains of adolescents than in brains of mature adults. Specifically, does experimenting with nicotine, alcohol, marijuana, and other drugs during adolescence affect normal brain development in any significant way? Does initiation of drug use in adolescence affect future cognitive or emotional function for better or worse in ways that later initiation of drug use does not? Does early use make teens more likely to develop addiction either in adolescence or later in life? And if there are adverse effects, are they dependent on the dose of the drug or pattern of use?

A beginning answer is that adolescent brains in animals do respond differently than adult brains to some drugs.[38] We know, for example, that high doses of drugs cause damage in the adolescent rodent brain that may be permanent.[39] This finding confirms what we have observed over many years in human beings with addiction: high doses of drugs for a prolonged period may cause permanent brain damage.

But the answer to many of the more subtle questions is that we don't know . . . yet. The basic science research on isolated cell preparations, brain slices, or on animal models is generating data that pose as many new questions as they provide answers. Some of the results are so interesting and suggestive of previously unknown actions of drugs on the brain's structure and function that it is tempting to extrapolate these findings to humans. Dr. H. Scott Swartzwelder, a research scientist studying drug effects on animal brains at the U.S. Department of Veterans' Affairs and Duke University, advises us that, when looking at current research evidence, we should "translate it to the human sphere cautiously."[40] He goes on to say that human and rat brains are more similar, especially in the more primitive brain structures such as the hippocampus, than we might like to think, but our daily life experiences and the reflective cognitive abilities that humans bring to bear on their lives are significantly more complex than those of a rodent. With that caveat, let's look at what scientists have discovered.

Studies in animal models, typically rats or mice, show that the adolescent rodent brain does behave differently than the adult rodent brain when exposed to psychoactive drugs, either through acute intoxication or chronic exposure.[41] The data for the effects of alcohol are particularly robust because different research methods—animal behavior, brain imaging, and electrophysiological studies—have corroborated similar findings.[42] We shall first explore the effects of alcohol and then discuss the more preliminary findings with nicotine, cocaine, and cannabinoids.

Alcohol at high doses, particularly in a binge pattern of use, can impede or interrupt a rodent's normal neurogenesis, the process of forming new brain cells.[43] This toxic effect is dose-dependent, with higher doses decreasing neurogenesis by as much as 99 percent[44] and may continue for at least two days beyond the binge.[45] While alcohol also blocks neurogenesis in adult rat brains,[46] different areas are affected in adolescent versus adult rodent brains.[47] At the cellular level, alcohol may disrupt electrical signaling and receptor activity in adolescent rodent brains, changes that may persist into adulthood.[48] These toxic effects of alcohol may occur without any evidence of alteration in the animal's behavior or performance. More recent imaging studies of human adolescents with alcohol use disorders also show changes in brain structure and function without any manifest differences in behavior, in comparison to adolescent controls.[49]

So, you may say, if adolescents continue to behave and perform normally despite these cellular changes, perhaps the changes are not significant or occur only with very high doses of alcohol. In fact, many animal studies use amounts of alcohol that exceed typical human use of alcohol. As an example, the author, a 54 kilogram woman, would need to down thirty-two glasses of wine daily for three to seven days and then receive an injection of 300 milligrams of absolute alcohol to consume as much alcohol as rats received in one study of acute responses to alcohol.[50] In trying to find a threshold amount, one researcher found that both adult and adolescent rats given 0.5 milligram of alcohol per kilogram of body weight daily, about the equivalent of two drinks daily, showed no difficulty in acquiring spatial memory, but at 2.5 milligrams per kilogram (about ten drinks daily), both the adolescent and adult rats were similarly impaired.[51]

In response to acute alcohol intoxication, adolescent rodents are less affected physically, but more impaired in cognitive function, than adult rodents. Young adolescent rats appear particularly sensitive to the activating effects of low-dose alcohol.[52] The rowdiness of teenage friends socializing and drinking (illegally) in a park comes to mind. After exposure to similar amounts of alcohol, adolescent rats are less sedated and recover their ability to stand upright sooner than adult counterparts and at higher serum alcohol levels.[53] Adolescent rats cleared alcohol from their blood more rapidly than adult rodents and recovered more quickly from hangover effects, demonstrating less anxiety and more rapid return to social activity.[54] Several researchers found that intoxicated adolescent rats had more difficulty acquiring spatial memory (e.g., finding their way through a maze) than intoxicated adult rats.[55] Another study showed that adolescent and adult rats exposed to alcohol performed equally well on tests of spatial memory but used different parts of their brains.[56] Although spatial memory is impaired by acute intoxication, other aspects of memory appear unaffected.[57] In contrast, other research showed that male rats exposed to high chronic doses of alcohol as adolescents performed better on a spatial memory test as adults than rats without alcohol exposure as adolescents and also were more efficient in self-administering alcohol by pressing a bar.[58]

Given the opportunity, adolescent rats will self-administer more alcohol than adults, in both social and isolated circumstances.[59] Overall, adolescent rats rapidly develop tolerance to the effects of acute, binge, and chronic alcohol exposure.[60] Female adolescent mice exposed to "binge" drinking had significantly increased alcohol intake as adults.[61]

While adolescent rats are less sensitive than adult rats to alcohol, which is a sedative, they appear to be more sensitive to the stimulants nicotine and cocaine than adult rats. After two weeks of nicotine infusion, both adolescent and adult rats have demonstrated an upregulation of nicotine receptors, suggesting increasing sensitivity to nicotine.[62] Adolescent rats previously exposed to cocaine had an increased locomotor response when rechallenged with cocaine.[63] Adult rats exposed to nicotine as adolescents showed increased sensitization to nicotine compared with nicotine-naive adults.[64] These studies suggest that adolescents are more sensitive to the effects of stimulants (nicotine, cocaine) than adults and therefore might develop addiction at lower levels of drug use, an observation not lost on the marketing departments of tobacco companies. In contrast, the rapid tolerance to and recovery from the sedative effects of alcohol in adolescent rats might reinforce increased alcohol use. Without the negative effects of alcohol to act as a brake on consumption, adolescents would be more likely than adults to use more alcohol. The definitive patterns of adolescent rodent responses to different drugs and the implications for drug use as adults will require more research, but there is clear evidence to indicate that adult and adolescent rodent brains react differently to acute exposures to alcohol and other drugs.[65]

The long-term effects of heavy drug use by adolescent rodents are more worrisome. Consumption of alcohol, whether coerced or voluntary, by male adolescent rats appears to lead to increased alcohol consumption at a later age.[66] Adolescent exposure to alcohol as the only available fluid diminished most adult rodents' ability to perform certain cognitive tasks (although 5 percent showed improved performance).[67] Similarly, adult rats exposed to binge dosing of alcohol as adolescents had more problems with working memory following an alcohol challenge than did rats first exposed to binge dosing as adults.[68] In contrast, the stimulants nicotine and cocaine used in rats during their adolescence improved their performance on some cognitive tasks as adults.[69]

Adult rats that had been exposed to alcohol or stimulants (nicotine, cocaine, methylphenidate) during adolescence demonstrated increased interest in or response to some addictive drugs than adult rats without adolescent exposure to alcohol and stimulants.[70] Adolescent rats pretreated with cannabinoids, compared with control adolescent rats, appeared to develop increased tolerance not only to cannabinoids but also morphine, cocaine, and amphetamine as they grew up.[71] These studies suggest that heavy drug use in adolescence primes the rodent for increased use of or tolerance to the same or another drug in adulthood. As we shall discover in the next section, data from the social sciences confirm similar patterns in our adolescent children.

A key question for concerned parents and policy makers remains unanswered. We still do not know at what point teens' experimentation with drug use makes chronic harmful use or drug addiction more likely than an eventual moderation to lower-risk use. Nor do we know how much drug use in itself is the crucial issue, or how much increased personal vulnerability due to family genetics or to earlier childhood experiences is the critical variable in developing harmful drug use or dependence at any age. I am not talking here of the potentially lethal effects of intoxication itself or in combination with cars and excessive speed, which can occur with the first or any instance of experimentation with drugs. Keeping our children safe while they learn to keep themselves safe is paramount. The focus here is on adolescent development, not just the brain but the whole person, in relation to drug use.

Adolescence: Developing Brain, Maturing Person

The science of developmental psychology allows us to approach adolescent development by observing the whole person within his environment. To study teenagers' initiation of drug use, our first questions might be: At what age do we need to start observing this person? And just what are we looking for? And whom should we ask?

In a landmark observational study, L. Alan Sroufe, Irving B. Harris Professor of Child Psychology at the Institute of Child Development and adjunct professor of psychiatry at the University of Minnesota, and his colleagues from the University of Minnesota followed 180 children born into poverty from birth through childhood and adolescence to adulthood.[72] Over thirty years, they made direct observations of these children and their environments. "We examined parenting, peer relationships, temperament, and cognitive functioning, and we examined the interplay of all these factors age by age in detail, beginning at the beginning."[73] The researchers interviewed the children, their parents and caregivers, teachers, peers and intimate friends, and they assessed these children with a comprehensive battery of psychological tests multiple times. The focus of the study was threefold: (1) to understand what experiences led to and might predict competent functioning or, conversely, maladaptive behavior as an adolescent or young adult; (2) to explain the combinations of conditions that led some children to be resilient and others to have problems, and most important; (3) to understand "the very nature and process of development."[74]

Statistical analyses of the large data set in the Minnesota study enabled Sroufe to describe the plasticity of the development of the person. Like neuroscientists looking at the brain's function and connectivity, these psychologists are interested in the child's emotional and cognitive organization and function and the patterns of behavioral adaptation. Some early variables were strong but not absolute predictors of later outcomes: strong infant attachment to the mother or primary caregiver indicated positive competence from early childhood through adolescence, whereas a history of physical abuse when evaluated statistically was always associated with negative predictions.[75] Early predictors were mitigated by more recent developments and environmental forces. An adolescent's level of competence was built on, but not determined by, early experiences.

The most salient developmental issue for adolescents, according to Sroufe, is individuation, which subsumes autonomy with connectedness, identity, and competence with peers, school, and work.[76] A combination of positive early experience, middle childhood peer competence, and maternal support of the child in grades one to three predicted adolescent social competence in 69 percent of the subjects.[77]

How does the initiation of alcohol and drug use fit in? Earlier studies indicate that those teens who experiment with alcohol or marijuana appear to be more psychologically healthy than adolescents who either abstain or engage in heavy drug use.[78] In reviewing the data in his seventy-year prospective observation of two cohorts of young men, Dr. George Vaillant remarked that "capacity for sustained moderate drinking seems correlated with positive mental health" and "may be associated with good social skills and capacity to play."[79] Teens experimenting with marijuana manifested better interpersonal relations and less subjective distress at ages seven, eleven, and eighteen than either the frequent marijuana users or the abstainers.[80] In contrast to supportive parenting noted for the experimenter group, mothers of the other two groups appeared overly concerned with their children's performance while being less supportive and more hostile. For the frequent drug users, their relatively maladaptive patterns of behavior preceded their initiation of marijuana.[81] Other worrisome teen behaviors, in particular risky sexual behavior and association with deviant peers, were significantly predicted by negative experiences in early childhood and at age thirteen.[82] How much of the significant association among these maladaptive behaviors can we ascribe to similar early predictors, and how much to the effect of one current risky behavior on another or something else entirely? Using data from the Minnesota study, Drs. Jessica Siebenbruner, Michelle Englund, and their colleagues identified several developmental antecedents to substance use patterns in late adolescence.[83] Of the 176 participants aged seventeen and one-half years, over 70 percent were either "experimenters" with drugs (65 adolescents) or "at risk" users (63 adolescents).[84] The only significant difference between these groups was increased parental monitoring in the experimenter group, primarily in terms of clear parental expectations and good communication between parents and adolescents.[85] Compared with the experimenters, the abstainers had experienced more maternal hostility at ages two to three and one-half years and demonstrated more internalizing behavior (anxiety, depression, fear of making mistakes) at age sixteen. The alcohol abusers were more likely to be male, to have manifested externalizing behavior (aggression, defiance, delinquency) at ages six and sixteen, and to have a history of less parental monitoring than the experimenters.

Between ages nineteen and twenty-three, the patterns of alcohol use started to shift, most likely reflecting the cohort becoming of legal drinking age. About one-third continued to be heavy drinkers, but alcohol initiation by abstainers at age nineteen increased the pool of moderate drinkers from 44 to about 60 percent,[86] suggesting that moderate to heavy alcohol use was normative behavior for this age group. Heavy alcohol use at age sixteen by men predicted continued moderate to heavy use and alcohol use disorders (AUD) at age twenty-eight. There was a similar but not statistically significant trend for women. On the other hand, fewer than 10 percent of all heavy users at age nineteen had AUDs by age twenty-eight.

Other than heavy drinking at age sixteen, what other developmental issues differentiate the twenty-six-year-old heavy users and twenty-eight-year-olds with AUD from their moderate-drinking peers? Data from the Minnesota study suggest several individual and parental factors. Behaviors such as aggression, defiance, and nervousness in childhood correlate with heavier alcohol use and AUDs, implying that both sets of behavior may reflect underlying emotional dysregulation and difficulties with control.

Parental hostility, neglect, or abuse in early childhood appears to be associated with later conduct disorder issues including externalizing behaviors.[87] Increased drinking among their mothers, described by study participants at age sixteen, also influenced heavy drinking in early adulthood. Dr. Englund succinctly summarizes: "Perhaps a genetic predisposition to alcohol disorders coupled with poor parenting leading to behavioral dysregulation in childhood together with a perception of heavy alcohol use as acceptable behavior may place individuals on a pathway towards heavier drinking in adolescence and into early adulthood."[88]

When interviewed again at age twenty-eight, just 7 percent of 161 participants met the criteria for AUD, but over 50 percent recalled symptoms in the prior ten years that met the criteria for a substance use disorder.[89] Data collected at ages nineteen and twenty-six for alcohol use show that the percentage of heavy alcohol drinkers at these ages was 32 (other drug use not included). This is a fascinating finding: over a roughly five-year span, between 30 and 40 percent of the group had matured from risky or problematic alcohol use patterns to light or moderate drinking. Did these subjects who had moderated their alcohol use have the same problem as the 7 percent that continued to have problems (i.e., met the criteria for AUD), or were there two different processes that appeared the same behaviorally but had different etiologies? The idea is intriguing, but the numbers in the subanalysis from the longitudinal Minnesota study are small, and more suggestive than definitive. Should future research confirm that there might be more than one explanation of adolescent drinking behavior, we may need to rethink our approaches to teenage substance use prevention and treatment.

We are left with the somewhat reassuring perspective that despite a 30 to 50 percent prevalence of apparent substance abuse behaviors in the late teens and early twenties, these disorders affect fewer than 10 percent of adults as they emerge from the turmoil of adolescence and early adulthood. But how many adolescents will have significant alterations of brain chemistry and function from experimenting with drugs? And for how many will these changes be permanent, beyond the brain's ability to compensate and repair itself? For those whose substance use problems do progress to addiction, the answer is many of them, as we shall learn in the next chapter. For the others, we do not know, but I would expect that a majority of adolescents experimenting with drugs do not suffer long-term health or psychological consequences. However, some children, because of genetic and environmental factors, are more vulnerable to the particular effects of drugs on the adolescent brain. Future research will help us identify those at highest risk. In the meantime, we will continue to debate the best ways to keep our children safe while encouraging them to explore and understand the world around them.

Low-Risk and Risky Alcohol Use: A Look at National Guidelines

The urge to try potentially addicting, mind-altering drugs is widespread. But what happens next? One way to approach this question is to look broadly at the patterns of drug use across American society. At any one time, about half of people twelve years of age and older (134 million) are current users (used in the past thirty days) of alcohol, and one-quarter

(68.2 million) use tobacco products, whereas fewer than 10 percent of that population (22 million) are using illicit drugs. For almost two-thirds of illicit drug users, that use is marijuana only.[90]

The degree of drug use covers a wide spectrum from abstinence (virtually no use) to daily excessive and harmful use. More Americans drink alcohol than use any other potentially dangerous addictive drug. Approximately one-third of Americans are abstinent from alcohol. Here abstinence is defined as no alcoholic drink in twelve or more months. At the other end of the spectrum are those with alcohol dependence or addiction. In between are those who drink but do not meet the criteria for addiction. These are the patients who ask me if their drinking is "normal."

HT, a twenty-nine-year-old graduate student in anthropology, comes in for a checkup. She tells me that she got married six months ago to a fellow graduate student, who is French. When I ask her about exercise, diet, and drug use, she notes she and her husband split a bottle of wine at dinner almost every night. Is this normal drinking?

BA, a seventy-five-year-old retired professor, has a martini before and two glasses of wine with his dinner, as he has for the last forty years. Is his drinking normal?

AW is a thirty-two-year-old mother of three children. Her father died of scarring of the liver (cirrhosis) due to his drinking. She knows that alcohol problems can run in families. Is it normal for her to have three to four drinks a week?

Normal refers to cultural norms—what is acceptable or expected within a particular group. These norms, based on customs and traditions, vary widely. All these people use alcohol in a way that is normative for their social group. What these patients are really asking me is whether their drinking is bad for their health. Safe or "low risk" drinking amounts are based on scientific evidence, albeit evidence interpreted through a particular culture's lens. HT's sharing a bottle of wine at dinner with her French husband is certainly normative within French tradition, but the guidelines from the National Institute on Alcohol Abuse and Alcoholism (NIAAA) would classify their behavior as "at risk" drinking.[91]

The NIAAA has based its guidelines for drinking alcohol on research data describing the relationships between the volume of alcohol consumed and various health conditions, such as hypertension, heart dis-

Table 1.1 NIAAA Recommended Low-Risk Drinking Limits for Healthy Adults

	Men up to age 65	Women (and men over age 65)
Daily	No more than 4 drinks in a day	No more than 3 drinks in a day
Weekly	No more than 14 drinks in a week	No more than 7 drinks in a week

Source: Adapted from U.S. National Institute on Alcohol Abuse and Alcoholism (2004).

Note: No use in risky situations (driving, pregnancy, certain medical conditions and medications). Depending on your health status, your doctor may advise you to drink less or abstain.

ease, cancers, and violence. The current recommendations (summarized in table 1.1) are the following: for women, no more than three drinks per occasion, no more than seven drinks weekly, and no use in a risky situation, such as operating heavy machinery, being pregnant, or taking medications that interact with alcohol; for men, no more than four drinks per occasion, no more than fourteen per week, and no use in a risky situation. People over age sixty-five are advised to limit their use to no more than seven drinks weekly and three per occasion.

Consumption of alcohol above three to four drinks daily increases the risk for heart disease, stomach, pancreas, and liver problems, cancers of the mouth, throat, and liver, sleep disturbances, and depression. This sustained heavy alcohol use may also cause dysfunction in other organ systems, such as the musculoskeletal, immune, and reproductive systems. A single instance of binge drinking may result in a fatal car crash. There is a very strong association between alcohol use and violence of all kinds, especially intimate partner abuse.

The group of people drinking at this "at-risk" or hazardous level comprises 15 to 20 percent of the population over twelve years. A significant subset of them will develop alcohol abuse and possibly dependence. A similar pattern is seen with users of other drugs; about 10 percent of them will develop abuse or dependence. With illicit drugs and nicotine, we are less aware of the people using the substance in an occasional "low risk" way. Some would argue that the illegal status of any drug makes all use "risky." While I agree that the unknown potency and impurity of illicit drugs and the possibility of arrest for drug possession can have negative consequences, there is no evidence from a medical perspective that the occasional use of small amounts of marijuana or an opioid is harmful. Because stimulants like amphetamines and cocaine may have acute toxic effects, including cardiac arrest and death, any casual use of them is risky. And of course, a person vulnerable to addiction will be at higher risk for problems whether a drug is legal or illicit.

The approximately 10 percent of people using drugs who develop and suffer addiction are the focus of the rest of this book. These people are our parents, children, brothers and sisters, cousins and grandparents, our colleagues at work, and our next-door neighbors. We will look at the changes in brain structure and function and the consequent changes in behavior that define their chronic illness. We will identify those most at risk for developing an addiction. We shall see how people manage and "live with" their addictions and review the contributions of medication and other treatment. Along the way, you will hear the stories of the people with addiction whom you met in the introduction.

TWO

SCIENCE OF ADDICTION

The term *addiction* conjures fearful images of deviant drug seekers who prey upon society for their own pleasure. This stereotype provokes intense negative emotions that overpower our reason and blind us to the facts. A large body of scientific research confirms that addiction is a disease of the brain. Chronic compulsive use of drugs can cause permanent changes in brain functioning. While trying to understand how addiction changes the brain, scientists have had to learn how the normal brain works. The unraveling of this mystery reads like a scientific thriller. For people suffering with addiction, the story is often more tragedy than thriller—repeated disappointments, failures, and losses, and the pain of a brain turned against itself. This chapter will integrate the scientific and human stories into a more coherent understanding of addiction.

The common, albeit stereotyped, images of addicted people are testimony to the pervasive influence of folk culture on our understanding of this illness. One common folk paradigm is that there are two populations, one of addicts and the other, the rest of us. You either have the disease of addiction, in which case you are most likely a "bum" to be avoided, or you don't. A dichotomy. As we discussed in the previous chapter, using addictive drugs is a learned behavior. Low-risk drug use, which is not a disease, and addiction are at opposite ends of a continuum. There are many heavy drinkers and drug users who never develop the pattern of compulsive behavior that defines addiction. They may have consequences from heavy use of drugs combined with poor judgment: motor vehicle crashes, falls, risky sexual encounters—what the American Psychiatric Society termed (until recently) "substance abuse."[1] Conversely, a small number of people who have used alcohol compulsively in the past do return to low-risk drinking as they mature and life circumstances change.[2]

The second folk myth is also an either-or conceptualization. At some point in the course of a person's addiction, he either abstains from the drug and recovers or continues on a progressive downhill course to death. According to Alcoholics Anonymous' (AA) oral tradition, this slide is inexorable. An addict would not be able to recover until he had progressed to a very severe stage of the illness, reached his "rock bottom" in the vernacular of AA.[3] Several research studies that have followed people for many years show that addiction has a more complicated and varied course.[4]

The Compulsion to Use

Compulsive behavior is the essence of addiction. At the heart of this chronic illness is a recurrent pattern of uncontrollable habitual behavior —usually the use of a drug, but other behaviors like compulsive gambling also fit the bill—despite known negative consequences.

There is ongoing debate about whether addictive behavior is *uncontrolled* or *uncontrollable*. *Addiction and Self-Control,* a new collection of essays from academic psychologists, neuroscientists, philosophers, economists, and legal experts, presents arguments for each side.[5] The issue is whether an addicted person has the agency (self-control) to prevent the neurological cascade from severe drug cravings (desires) to the automatic behaviors leading to drug use. As a clinician working with addicted patients, I see this as a false dichotomy. The intensity of desires is on a continuum, as is the ability to control actions related to them. Like adolescents, addicted people need to develop the emotional and cognitive maturity to control their desires and behaviors. It takes years for someone to learn enough skills to manage the intensity of their impulses and the subsequent behaviors; this is the process of adolescence and also of recovery. For those whose addiction is in remission, a major personal loss (sudden death of a spouse) plus an emotional vulnerability may precipitate an uncontrollable brief lapse to drug use. A prolonged relapse in someone who has demonstrated the ability to manage her addiction is more probably uncontrolled behavior.

The negative consequences of this behavior can be as private as worsening self-esteem with every relapse. Whenever Linda describes herself as "such a failure because I've relapsed ten times," I counter with the observation that returning to treatment for the eleventh time shows incredible perseverance. Certainly, many of the painful consequences of addiction are hidden behind closed doors: a distrustful wife feeling betrayed by her spouse's relapse, the teenager who won't invite friends to his house because his mother may be drunk again. What the public sees—the fatal car crash or the increased number of neighborhood break-ins by addicted people desperate for cash to buy drugs—is only the tip of the iceberg. As her addiction became more severe, Linda's compulsive behavior pattern engulfed her entire life so that she spent hours thinking about the drug, obtaining it, preparing it, using it, recovering from its use. Most addictions are devastating; others we can live with. Often the difference depends on the pharmacology of a particular drug, whether it is licit or illicit, and the circumstances of the addicted person's life. At first glance, addictive behaviors seem incomprehensible, alien, but many of us are more familiar with them than we might think.

Several years ago, at a workshop on addiction for legal aid attorneys, I tried to illustrate that point.

I stand at the podium of a law school amphitheater and look up at fifty or so lawyers and paraprofessionals. They peer down at me over coffee mugs, large Styrofoam cups labeled "The BIG ONE," lattes, and cappuccinos. "So," I say to break the ice, "I see that most of you have your drug of choice this morning." Slightly nervous laughter. "Let's talk about caffeine."

"How many of you don't use any caffeine?" A few hands are raised.

"Now, how about one or two cups of coffee or caffeinated sodas a day?" There's a rustling as a majority of people raise their hands.

"Three to six cups a day?" Perhaps a quarter of hands go up.

"More than six?" Audience members turn in their seats to see which of their colleagues will admit to drinking such an excessive amount of caffeine.

I push the discussion further. "That first cup of coffee is pretty important. Many people have their morning coffee ritual. Would anyone be willing to share their morning ritual?"

"Every morning I think about that first cup from the time I wake up until I get to my favorite Dunkin' Donuts. They don't even need to ask me what I want."

"My husband gets up before I do, so there's always this great smell of fresh coffee. Sometimes it's part of my dreams as I'm waking up. That first cup really starts my day."

"I set the timer on my coffee maker the night before, so it's all ready by the time my alarm clock goes off." A smattering of admiring applause.

"Sounds like that morning cup of coffee is pretty important. A lot of that has to do with how comforting habits can be for all of us." Now I want to know how much priority that morning coffee has in their lives. "How many of you would be a few minutes late for work to make sure you got that cup of coffee?"

Almost every hand goes up.

"How about ten minutes late?"

Only a few hands are raised.

"How many would make sure that you got your coffee before meeting with your boss for a performance review, even if getting your coffee would make you late?"

Uneasy gazes around the amphitheater, but no hands.

Caffeine is an addictive drug—but only mildly so. Our rituals of anticipating, preparing, and using caffeine are habits, a comfortable part of our daily routines. Caffeine may be important enough so that its use intrudes a bit into our daily obligations, but it doesn't overwhelm our responsibility to work or family. The organizing part of our brains, the prefrontal cortex, continues to exert its control over our desires and functioning. Nonetheless, as people with insomnia really have to have that fifth or sixth cup to get through the day, we are seeing caffeine addiction in action.

Recent research confirms that many of the apparently disparate theories to explain addiction actually relate to particular functions of different areas of the brain. Like the five blind men who discover an elephant and each is certain that the part of the elephant he touches describes the whole, scientists are discovering that addiction disrupts an extremely complicated, interconnected network of brain functions. Theories supported by current research encompass learning about drug rewards, increasing the motivation and salience of drugs, impaired decision making with decreased control over drug-related activities, increasingly rigid habitual behaviors, and the development of negative experiences and feelings that reinforce continued drug use. The evidence implies that the dysregulation of specific brain networks involved in reward-related behaviors can account for the typical addictive behaviors of compulsive drug use, impaired self-control, and lack of behavioral flexibility.[6] These are my patients' lived experiences. Linda, who now, in recovery, knows and demonstrates that her children are the most precious thing in her life, spent two years living on the street injecting drugs while family members cared for her very young daughters.

Recent addiction research is clear: one factor in the compulsive use of drugs is a decreased ability to control drug use. Experiments from many areas of science—work at the molecular and cellular level, research using animal models of addiction, neuroimaging that allows us to visualize the human brain in action, clinical observations—corroborate this hypothesis. How does addiction to powerful drugs like nicotine, cocaine, alcohol, or heroin create this uncontrollable compulsion? The cross-fertilization of recent neuroscience research on addiction and well-established psychological conditioning studies has advanced our understanding of the brain's normal reward functions.

For a species to survive, its members need to live long enough to mate and ensure the survival of their young. Over millions of years, the brain has evolved to ensure that the most basic survival needs—being safe, eating, mating, and nurturing the young—are experienced as rewarding or pleasurable. We find that we enjoy or "like" these essential survival activities, often unaware that the pursuit of these pleasures is no frivolous endeavor. Because we are likely to repeat behaviors with pleasurable outcomes, these activities become self-reinforcing.[7] This positive reinforcement is necessary for some aspects of memory and learning.[8]

Let's break down this experience of reward. First, we need to have a pleasurable experience, a rewarding activity that we like enough to want to experience it again. The pleasurable stimulus is "liked" because it makes doing certain things feel better.[9] Our own inner drives of hunger and thirst, or stressful states, may increase our motivation to seek these rewards. Not only do I like the taste of freshly baked molasses clove cookies, but if I am hungry, I will "want" them even more. My internal state of hunger has increased my motivation to find the cookie jar and enhanced the incentive value of the cookie reward.

Usually with fresh-baked cookies, it is the smell that triggers the wanting, but it could be the cookie jar, a cue without any characteristics of the cookie. Environmental cues are often strongly motivating; they activate an intense desire and initiate a behavioral response before we experience the reward. These behaviors can be very complex, requiring practice and flexibility to achieve the reward. As an animal becomes more effective and efficient in performing a sequence of behaviors like searching for food, these responses become automatic or habitual,[10] and the neural pathways to achieve them are deeply ingrained.

As I watch the biggest, fattest squirrel that lives in the old sugar maple tree outside my kitchen window, these concepts begin to make sense. This squirrel has been around for several years, chasing other squirrels away from its food source. By November, its cheeks and belly are so fat that I don't know how it manages to leap six feet to the top of the fence. The squirrel has clearly figured out where to go for the best, most plentiful food—and that is underneath the bird feeder.

Associated areas of the squirrel's brain (fig. 2.1), the mesolimbic and prefrontal cortex (PFC), have formed memories associated with the birdseed reward, cues such as the twittering presence of sparrows. The memories of the correct sequence of behaviors to get from his nest in the sugar maple to this plentiful source of food are stored in the adjacent dorsal striatum. Whenever the birds come to feed, the squirrel scurries down to the feeder, just waiting for bits of seed to rain down around him. As this pattern of behavior solidifies, it becomes a "no-brainer" habit: a reward-related cue triggers an action with minimal, if any, monitoring from higher brain centers. This squirrel's ability to fulfill its needs efficiently and effectively gives it a clear survival advantage over its scrawny neighbors. The animal must also adapt to changes in the environment and prioritize which of its needs to act upon. Two areas in the more cognitive parts of the brain (the orbitofrontal complex [OFC] and the cingulate cortex) monitor changes in sensory stimuli and direct adaptive mecha-

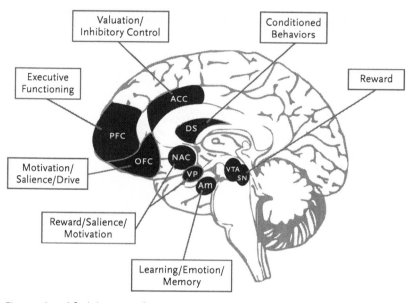

Fig. 2.1 Simplified diagram of cortico-mesolimbic (reward) system.

PFC	prefrontal cortex	VP	ventral pallidum
ACC	anterior cingulate cortex	Am	amygdala
OFC	orbitofrontal cortex	VTA	ventral tegmental area
DS	dorsal striatum	SN	substantia nigra
NAC	nucleus accumbens		

Adapted from National Institute on Drug Abuse.

nisms.[11] In adults with mature brains, these cognitive centers compare the benefits and risks of this pleasurable experience against many other priorities, exerting a "top down" control over behaviors.[12] So, while the squirrel may be enjoying a shower of birdseed, the sight of an approaching dog will change the priorities to safety over food, as it leaps up a tree trunk out of harm's way.

I use the example of the squirrel to underscore that the brain's reward mechanism governs normal survival behaviors. In fact, the rewarding part of this pathway is active primarily when the brain is learning that it likes certain outcomes. This experience of liking occurs in different networks of the brain (cortico-mesolimbic region) than the experience of wanting (OFC) and the initiation and maintenance of actions to fulfill these wants (dorsal striatum).[13]

What this means is that the pleasure of anticipation (wanting and desiring) and the pleasure of liking are separate brain functions. This should not be a surprise to most people. For me, looking forward to a beautiful day of hiking, informed by memories of clear October weather and views of beautiful New England foliage, will get me to the mountains. Once there, the reality may be an overcast sky with a chilling wind. My desire for a usually pleasant experience has resulted in my being cold and miserable.

Bill, after two years of abstinence, wears his frustration and anger on his face. "I used," he says, sounding disgusted. "I hate what drugs have done to me; I know I don't want to use. Even when I have a needle in my arm, I don't want to use."

"What happened?" I ask.

"My brother told me I have to move out, because his girlfriend is moving in. He won't even let me sleep on his couch till I find another place. I'll be homeless again."

"And then?"

"It felt like my life was falling apart again, and I started thinking about using. I knew I needed to get to an AA meeting. So I called a buddy to get a ride. On the way, he offered me some dope [heroin]. I'm so pissed he did this to me; he had told me he was clean. Suddenly, getting high just seemed to make more sense than anything else. I couldn't wait to forget all the shit in my life and feel a lot better. All I wanted was to get high."

"Did it help?"

"I didn't even get a high. By the time I was shooting up, I already felt like such an asshole. I didn't like what I was doing; I fucked up again."

Bill had tried to do the right thing. He was on a medication that blocked the effects of heroin, so that there was no positive reinforcement for injecting heroin. But by then it was already too late. He had recognized that his despair about being homeless again made him vulnerable to relapse and had made the safe decision to go to a meeting. Blindsided by the unexpected immediate access to heroin, his intense cravings overpowered his judgment and led to the outcome of feeling even worse about himself. But he didn't continue to inject heroin, despite his negative mind-set. This was progress for Bill.

The research data that underlie the simple vignettes of the squirrel's behavior and of Bill's brief lapse indicate a far more complicated system, involving interconnected circuits and feedback loops, than the linear one I have described. Several different chemicals transmit signals from one area to another. From the molecular level to neuronal circuits connecting different parts of the brain, scientists have made huge advances in understanding specific interactions between functional areas of the brain.[14] But how these elegant processes fit together as a whole still eludes us.

Pieces of the Puzzle

Addictive drugs, other rewards, and internal or environmental cues act directly on the cortico-mesolimbic reward system, stimulating dopamine directly or other transmitters that then influence dopamine activity. Rewarding stimuli first activate two areas of the brain (the ventral tegmental area and the substantia nigra) that initiate the dopamine pathway. This pathway or, as it turns out, several pathways are essential elements of the reward process. In the mid-1960s, two addiction scientists, Dr. Vincent Dole and Dr. Marie Nyswander from Rockefeller University in New York, hypothesized from their studies of heroin addiction that dopamine was the primary neurotransmitter in reward and addiction.[15] Neuroscientists are still unraveling its complex functions.

It turns out that the most common explanation for addiction, that dopamine mediates the pleasure of using drugs and the unpleasant effects of stopping use (withdrawal from drugs), is a misleading simplification.[16] The positive rewards of drug use and negative effects of stopping use are certainly involved in the reinforcement for continuation of early drug use, but they do not explain the phenomenon of addiction.

One of the more widely accepted theories is that the dopamine reward pathway represents a process of expectation, learning, memory formation, and relearning, rather than one of pleasure and pain. Dopamine is not involved with the neural circuits that encode the specifics of a reward experience—the enticing odor of that freshly baked cookie or the gorgeous harmonies in Mahler's fourth symphony. One of dopamine's functions is to signal whether an experience is better than, worse than, or the same as predicted, irrespective of its content.

Let's go back to the fat squirrel, which has certain expectations about the birdseed it will find under the feeder. This time when the twittering sparrows appear, the squirrel hops down to the feeder only to discover that it is empty and the birds are just bickering, not eating. No food. In this scenario, the experience is worse than predicted, and the squirrel may look elsewhere for food. Two days later, the squirrel hears the birds and again hops down to the feeder. The usual prediction that there will be plenty of food has been tempered slightly by the most recent experience with the empty feeder. The squirrel finds the familiar shower of birdseed, so it resumes the usual feeding pattern. The experience is just like the squirrel's expectation; no new learning has occurred. A find of intact sunflower seeds strewn on the ground the next day is clearly better than predicted. The squirrel returns to the feeder more frequently. When an experience is better than predicted, dopamine levels in the nucleus accumbens, amygdala, and PFC increase. Conversely, if the experience is worse than predicted, the amount of dopamine decreases. If the experience is just as predicted, there is no change in the baseline dopamine level. Observations like these in the more controlled environment of the laboratory have led to the "prediction error" hypothesis. New learning leading to changed behavior in pursuit of a reward occurs only if the reality is different—better or worse—from the prediction.[17] This means that a person taking her first drinks of alcohol already has an expectation of intoxication from the vicarious memories of her drinking friends' stories or the culture around her. In the nucleus accumbens, higher dopamine levels appear to increase motivation to reach that particular reward.

Over time, a cue indicating that the rewarding outcome is nearby, rather than the reward itself, triggers reward-seeking behavior. Our squirrel needs only to hear the twittering birds to start seeking the reward goal of birdseed. It does not need the rewarding taste of the first bite. A simpler example involves the automatic behavior of Pavlov's dog. After becoming used to hearing a bell ring shortly before he received a sausage treat, the dog would begin to salivate at the sound of the bell whether or not a sausage was finally forthcoming. Salivation is an autonomic response and occurs without any conscious behavioral response from the dog. Psychologists call this phenomenon of a stimulus followed by autonomic response "classic" conditioning.

The squirrel's response to the stimulus of the birds is more sophisticated. In order to receive the reward of birdseed, it has had to perform a conditioned sequence of behaviors—leaving its nest, going to the bird feeder, sitting under it until the seeds fall, then picking them up off the ground and eating them. This "instrumental conditioning," a stimulus followed by a behavioral response, represents learned behavior. Professor Wolfram Schultz from the Department of Anatomy at the University of Cambridge, UK, explains further that "three factors govern conditioning, namely contiguity, contingency, and prediction error."[18] We have already discussed prediction error. Contiguity refers to the temporal relationship between the stimulus and reward; for effective conditioning, this relationship should be a matter of seconds. Using a rapid-acting drug and the fastest method to get a drug to the brain (smoking nicotine or cocaine) is contiguity in action. Contingency implies that the reward will occur more frequently in response to a unique stimulus. If that stimulus is meeting one's drug dealer, the addicted person will experience intense craving even before the drug has changed hands. If the sparrows twittered all the time whether they were feeding or not, their noise would no longer be a specific cue for the squirrel to seek the reward of birdseed. The contiguity and contingency of a stimulus and response enable and reinforce the conditioned learning.

If a cue that the reward is at hand stimulates reward-seeking behavior, just what is the animal responding to? Certainly, not the pharmacological effect of a drug not yet taken. The animal needs to have a memory of the reward associated with the cue that in itself does not have any of the physical characteristics of the reward—its taste, dimensions, color. Rather, the cue triggers memory and expectation of how rewarding the goal will be. For an addicted person, persistent maladaptive memories, probably aggrandized by drug-induced distortions of signaling mechanisms, perpetuate compulsive drug seeking and use.[19] The degree of satisfaction a reward delivers is a function both of properties intrinsic to the reward and of factors specific to the host and the environment.[20] For instance, if the squirrel has just finished a meal of acorns and is feeling satiated, it may perceive the sunflower seeds as less rewarding even though the actual characteristics of the seeds have not changed. The animal may have an increased "wanting" of the rewards triggered by the cue of twittering sparrows without a change in its "liking" of it. This distinction between the "liking" of the reward itself and the "wanting" of the reward from memories triggered by a cue signifies a major development in our conceptual understanding of addiction. Research scientists are working to confirm all the steps in this hypothesis, but for a clinician this conceptualization explains a common observation of addictive behavior. An addicted patient will declare emphatically that he does not like or plan to use drugs anymore and then leave my office, unexpectedly see his drug dealer across the street, and succumb to powerful craving, "wanting," for the drug. Bill, after a few months' remission on buprenorphine/naloxone (Suboxone) addiction treatment, was baffled by his behavior: "I don't know why I keep using drugs. I don't like the experience. I don't even want to use, but somehow I do."

Rephrasing this apparent contradiction in neurophysiological terms suggests that the activations of neuronal cells in the "wanting" part of the brain represent expectations of the reward.[21] As a reward is more predictably expected through learning trials, the orbitofrontal cortex and amygdala show increased activation. In a confirmatory experiment, rats with lesions of the amygdala are unable to execute the sequence of behaviors to obtain a cocaine reward, whereas they are able to self-administer cocaine if it is right in front of them.[22] These behaviors suggest that reward seeking may have more to do with the anticipation of reward than with the liking of it. Schultz hypothesizes that the three-way switch of increased, decreased, or no change in dopamine in response to the prediction error may actually function in a modulated and more subtle way, much like the rheostat on a light switch.

Other neurotransmitters play key roles in the reward-processing system. Gamma amino butyric acid, the neurotransmitter most involved in responses to alcohol, influences dopamine's effects. Its inhibitory action tempers the magnitude of the dopamine response to drugs. Another transmitter, glutamate, appears to interact with dopamine in the process of learning.[23] Martha discovered that Klonopin could activate these processes as well as, or better than, vodka. Changes in dopamine levels mimic stressful situations by increasing corticotropin releasing factor (CRF) in the amygdala. CRF, by targeting other hormones, triggers physiologic responses to stress—increased alertness, rapid heartbeat, sweating, and anxiety.

As the outcome of an animal's trial behavior becomes more predictable, the behavior becomes more habitual. Now the squirrel scampers down the tree to the bird feeder not so much because it likes birdseed but rather because the twittering of the birds triggers automatic habitual behavior to seek birdseed. Now that there is nothing new to learn, the prefrontal cortex, the top-down control area of the brain, is less involved. Once the squirrel's brain has identified a cue and learned behaviors to obtain the reward, finding food is an automatic, habitual activity.[24] The brain is free to solve more pressing survival problems.

The elegant role of this pathway in mankind's survival skills is sabotaged by addictive drugs. All these drugs directly or indirectly elevate the level of dopamine in the mid- and forebrain. With increased dopamine, every episode of drug use is experienced as "better than expected," even though the reality may be mostly negative. Dr. Steven Hyman comments, "Mechanisms that evolved to motivate survival behaviors, the pursuit of natural rewards, are usurped by the potent and abnormal dopamine signal produced by addictive drugs."[25] They disrupt and overwhelm the delicate balance of the neuronal circuits so that to Linda, in her late teens, obtaining and taking drugs became as automatic as normal survival behaviors.

We need to examine the pharmacology of these drugs to understand how they increase dopamine levels in the brain.[26] The stimulants cocaine and amphetamine are the most straightforward. Their actions are very similar to those of dopamine, so that they can act directly on dopamine receptors to increase the amount of dopamine released and to disrupt the uptake of dopamine back into the neuron (fig. 2.2). Instead of the usual clearing of dopamine back into the dispensing cell in preparation for release with another stimulus, dopamine continues to flood the synapse (the space between two communicating neurons), immediately magnifying the effects of the person's own endogenous dopamine. Nicotine, a

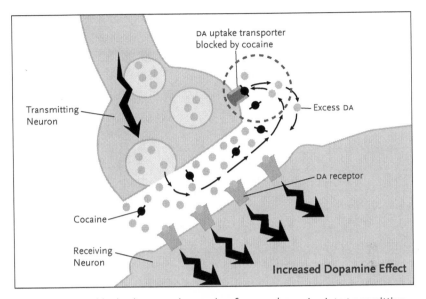

Fig. 2.2 Cocaine blocks the normal reuptake of excess dopamine into transmitting cells, resulting in flooding of the dopamine receptors in receiving neurons and increasing the dopamine effect. DA—dopamine. Adapted from the National Institute on Drug Abuse.

weaker stimulant, mimics the neurotransmitter acetylcholine at acetylcholine receptors, which in turn activate dopamine neurons.

Sedatives have a more circuitous route. Opioids bind to *mu* and *kappa* opiate receptors in the brain. These receptors are part of our body's opiate system of endorphins, which mediate pain and other bodily sensations. The ventral tegmental area at the beginning of the dopamine pathway has many *mu* receptors. When flooded with heroin or the potent painkiller oxycodone, these receptors trigger the release of large amounts of dopamine.

Alcohol affects a number of different neurotransmitters, primarily glutamate and gamma amino butyric acid. This system inhibits dopamine activities; alcohol, by inhibiting this system, causes an increase in available dopamine. As an analogue of glutamate, alcohol blocks the n-methyl-d-aspartate receptors; the excess glutamate leads to an increase in dopamine.

The natural neurotransmitter anandamide has properties mimicked by marijuana. Marijuana acts at some of the anandamide receptors in the brain (CB1 receptors), increasing their effect on dopamine neurons.

The bottom line is that every addictive drug studied increases the amount of dopamine released by the brain. The elevated dopamine levels signal a positive prediction error; every drug experience becomes "better than expected."[27] A positive prediction error drives a person to repeat the experience more and more frequently, rapidly reinforcing drug-taking behaviors. Initially part of a flexible response that can reorganize behaviors when inputs change, the repetition of these experiences leads to rigid, ingrained behaviors. The OFC, which helps to form and value associated memories, is involved in modifying cellular responses if reinforcements change.[28] When the change is recurrent tidal waves of dopamine triggered by taking addictive drugs, the response at these sites is to decrease the number of dopamine D2 receptors and the amount of dopamine released.[29] Responses to natural pleasures are thus blunted. Over time the OFC loses the ability to prioritize among different rewards. Drug-associated motivation is so powerful that motivations toward natural rewards become undervalued. The only salient motivator is the drug itself or an associated cue.

Researchers at the National Institute on Drug Abuse demonstrated this phenomenon by showing a series of videos to two groups of young men: one, a group whose cocaine abuse had been in remission for twelve months; the other, a control group of healthy volunteers who had never taken cocaine. The brain activity of men in both groups was followed using functional magnetic resonance imaging. The first video, a nature film of wild animals, stimulated a small response in the midbrains of both groups; this experience was a little better than predicted, but not much. The next video depicted someone preparing and injecting cocaine. The cocaine group had a huge response, whereas the control group showed no increased activity in their midbrains. Subsequently, the groups watched an erotic video. The control group had a very robust response of increased activity in the midbrain; this experience was much better than predicted for them. But the midbrains of the cocaine abusers in remission responded with a small blip not much larger than their response to the wildlife video.[30] The cocaine users' midbrains showed significant, possibly permanent changes in function. Not only had these subjects given up cocaine; they manifested significantly less response to one of life's simple pleasures, sexual activity.

At the same time, the brain areas involved in inhibitory control and executive functioning, the anterior cingulate cortex and parts of the pre-frontal cortex (PFC), are less active in the addicted brain. New imaging studies of addicted people's brains show decreased or altered metabolism in the PFC and cingulate cortex[31] that occurs during intoxication and per-sists in chronic users. Many neural processes associated with the PFC are disrupted by addiction, including self-control and behavioral monitoring, emotional regulation, motivation, attention, insight, learning and mem-ory, decision making, and salience attribution.[32] There is no question that an addict's decreased control over drug-taking activities has a physiologic basis. As Bill's behavior illustrated, these changes in an addicted person's limbic function could explain the irresistible salience of a drug cue even after months of abstinence and the difficulty of controlling drug-taking behavior once it has been initiated.[33] Not only does addiction overvalue the benefits and undervalue the costs of drug use; it may also disrupt the decision-making process and impair addicted people's ability to make ap-propriate, self-beneficial decisions.[34] For Larry and Delia, only a few years out of adolescence, this effect has been particularly difficult to overcome.

The brain has the capacity to adapt to changing stimuli by changing its own function and structure. This plasticity of brain tissue makes the brain susceptible to powerful new stimuli and may also allow it to re-vert toward normal. We know this is true in children, whose developing brains are very malleable. Neuroimaging studies, like the one just de-scribed, demonstrate plasticity at a circuit or system level. What are the mechanisms at the cellular and transmitter levels that allow the brain to respond like this? What makes this plasticity possible?

A couple of general principles may be helpful here. Over time, increas-ing or decreasing the amount of an input stimulus to a cell will change that cell's output. Some changes occur on the cell surface, others in the cell's interior (cytoplasm) or cell nucleus. In response to a stronger input stimulus, many cells will initially increase their capacity to handle the stimulus by increasing the number of cell surface receptors for that input. Scientists use the term "upregulation" to describe this cellular adapta-tion to increased input. With persistent excessive stimulus, the converse occurs; cells will "downregulate" the number of receptors and other in-tracellular mechanisms below their original levels in an attempt to compensate for the overstimulus. When the excessive neurotransmitter input returns to normal levels, the cell may be too depleted or damaged to return to its normal output. While at first glance these cellular responses seem straightforward, consider an increased inhibitory stimulus that ultimately downregulates that cell or system. For example, drinking alcohol decreases the inhibitory effects of the GABA system on neurons in the prefrontal cortex that regulate impulsivity. Many of us would recognize the resulting disinhibition as characteristic of early alcohol intoxication.

To upregulate in response to a drug stimulus, the cell must recognize that more receptors are needed, find the blueprint for that particular receptor's protein in the cell's genome, manufacture these new receptors, and transport them to the cell surface. This process requires a series of chemical messengers that prompt the nuclear genetic material, deoxyribonucleic acid (DNA) and ribonucleic acid (RNA), to copy the instructions for the cell to manufacture the protein building blocks for the receptors. Addictive drugs can disrupt the cell's normal function permanently by affecting which genes are expressed. Several researchers have hypothesized that these changes in gene expression and subsequent changes in protein manufacture have an important role in memory storage.[35] Memories stored in the hippocampus have precise neural circuits that correspond to one particular behavior. In contrast to this targeted activity, addictive drugs bombard the dopamine neurons in the ventral tegmental area and alter the entire reward system.

Keep in mind that the theory that dopamine functions in learning and memory formation more than in pleasure and nonpleasure is just one of several hypotheses about how addictive drugs affect the brain. Well-known, respected addiction researchers have postulated other models of addiction. In 1997 George F. Koob, a physiologist at the Scripps Research Institute in La Jolla, California, and his coauthor Michel Le Moal from Bordeaux, France, coined the term the "dark side" of drug addiction to describe their hypothesis of an antireward system.[36] Since many biological systems have opposing processes that serve to balance and regulate function, they postulate that the brain's reward system is offset by an antireward system involving negative reinforcement and adverse emotional states.

In Koob and Le Moal's view of the addiction process, there is a three-stage cycle of "binge/intoxication," "withdrawal/negative affect," and "preoccupation/anticipation" that takes the addicted brain into a downward spiral. In the first stage, impulsive use and the acute reinforcing effects of addictive drugs cause excessive dopamine release, which overstimulates and dysregulates the reward system. As the addiction progresses to compulsive drug use, increasing dependence and repeated episodes of withdrawal provide negative reinforcement for discontinuing drug use—in other words, positive reinforcement for continuing drug use. Irritability, dysphoria, physical and emotional discomfort define the second stage, "withdrawal/negative affect." The neural systems involved in stress and pain, such as corticotropin releasing factor, norepinephrine, and dynorphin, come into play, causing the negative states of anxiety and irritability. The motivation for drug use is no longer the pleasurable feelings induced by increased dopamine but rather the unpleasant experience of anxiety and irritability common to states of acute withdrawal and prolonged use. They postulate that this negative dysregulation persists into prolonged abstinence and renders the addict more susceptible to relapse.[37] In this "preoccupation/anticipation" stage, neural circuits that increase craving are reactivated by drug use, drug cues, and stress.[38] The plasticity of the neural circuitry is key to the adaptations in this model and in the dopamine-learning model. Koob and Le Moal seem to be saying that the brain makes a maladaptive adjustment to drug use in an attempt to maintain normal reward functions—in the end making things worse. This model fits Martha's pattern of alcohol and Klonopin addiction. Meeting with her son when he was intoxicated and hostile toward her was a strong trigger for relapse. A mother's love, fear, and guilt felt too painful to contain; picking up a drink could deaden the negative emotions. These feelings, which she knew would still be there once her drug use was in remission, and the added humiliation of having relapsed again would slowly erode her initial hope and determination after treatment, making her increasingly vulnerable to another trigger.

Observations that some animal models become more sensitive to addictive drugs with prolonged use gave rise to the sensitization theory. While developing tolerance to some of a drug's effects, the rodent becomes more sensitive to some other effects. This increased sensitization has not been confirmed in other animal models but has been identified in human adolescents' early exposure to nicotine. Another theory, less well developed, is that an addict develops an increased sensitization to some aspects of a drug while developing tolerance to others.[39]

Addiction: Willful or Uncontrollable?

Is the compulsion to use addicting drugs a willful decision or an activity not completely under voluntary control? We have just learned that the brain may adapt to repetitive drug use by assigning an overwhelming salience to a drug-related cue or to the drug itself, so that other motivating priorities cannot contend with the wanting (craving) to use drugs. At the same time, the addicted brain appears to have decreased regulatory control over this behavior. Is this decreased self-control a product of the addicting process, or is this lack of control what gets people into trouble with addiction in the first place? Are people with addiction somehow unable to exert self-control? Is it because they choose not to? Are they responsible for what happens when they are addicted or somehow exonerated by the fact of their addiction? This is the crux of the matter.

We are treading on rough philosophical and scientific terrain here. The imaging studies of Volkow and her colleagues strongly suggest that the addicted brain is not able to assert its normal regulatory controls in the face of the overwhelming salience of wanting drugs. The neural processes that conduct sensory inputs to the neurons involved in performing behaviors do not appear to be subject to the dictates of conscious will or willpower.[40] In his provocative book *The Illusion of Conscious Will*, Dr. Daniel Wegner, professor of psychology at Harvard University, asks whether the process that humans experience as conscious will can exist outside the systems of neural circuits and, if so, where? He hypothesizes that what we experience as our will—I decided to buy some milk, so I went to the store—may in fact be the positive feeling evoked when our desires and actions are congruent with our values—coffee tastes better with milk, and milk is good for my health. Our experience of the synchrony between our behavior and what we value is pleasing; therefore we must have intended to perform this behavior. Further psychological and neurobiological research will eventually confirm or negate Dr. Wegner's reductionist hypothesis. The important point here is that the sensation of will exists within the same neurobiological processes that effect liking or wanting. From a scientific perspective, will is a product of neural circuitry responding to the effects of neurotransmitters triggered by stimuli from elsewhere in the brain or from the outside world.

A dilemma for society is the degree to which a person with an acute neurological dysfunction should be held accountable for her behavior. Consider these scenarios:

SB, the father with severe type 1 diabetes, needs to pick up his son after basketball practice. This is a fifteen-minute drive, but as usual, he checks his blood sugar level before leaving and takes his glucose tablets and snacks in the car in case his blood sugar drops to unsafe levels that could cause confusion or unconsciousness. Coming to a stoplight, he feels acutely lightheaded, clumsy, and confused. He tries to pull his car off the road but is so groggy he hits the car in front of him.

A young pregnant lawyer with a known seizure disorder is advised by her doctor not to drive, because of a very small chance that being pregnant might affect the control of her seizures. For the first six months she avoids driving and does not have any seizures. Then she cautiously resumes driving but, during a quick trip to a local store, she has a seizure and crashes her car.

At his twenty-fifth college reunion, an engineer with alcohol addiction in remission for fifteen years stops by to see his fraternity brothers. He has no intention of drinking and thinks he can handle the frisson of anticipation he feels. Surrounded by his buddies, the memories of how much fun they used to have drinking and laughing flood his brain with dopamine. He hasn't touched alcohol for over fifteen years; maybe one drink would be OK. Hours later he stumbles back to his car intoxicated and crashes his car on the way back to his hotel.

Each of these people had an acute brain dysfunction due to a chronic illness that led to uncontrolled behavior (severely low blood sugar, a seizure, an unintended lapse to dangerous alcohol intoxication) and a bad outcome (car crash.) Each one thought that the risk of harm related to his or her chronic disease was low. They are all responsible for the consequences of their decisions, but does society hold them equally blameworthy? I contend that the acute intense craving for a drug and the consequent automatic behaviors is as much an acute brain dysfunction as acute confusion from low blood sugar or an unexpected seizure, but I know many others would disagree.

The tendency for people to relapse to drug use after months or years in remission is one of the most damaging aspects of addiction, yet the drive to restart using drugs is often overwhelming. Where does that drive come from?

In the United States, we put a premium on self-control, personal discipline, and individual responsibility. If avoiding relapse were simply a matter of exerting one's will, then we Americans should have very low relapse rates. Emerging research suggests that relapse to drug use is initiated in parts of the brain beyond the reach of conscious choice. Sensory information associated with past use (e.g., the sight of a favorite drinking buddy, a certain Jimi Hendrix song, the pungent odor of marijuana smoke) cues memories in the OFC and nucleus accumbens of wanting drugs. These intense desires, relayed to the amygdala and dorsal striatum, trigger drug-seeking behaviors, even at a time when the person is consciously noting that he no longer likes the drug experience. The controls of the PFC are no match for the accelerating momentum to seek drugs.

Professor Wegner highlights this experience by quoting the main character in *The Reader*, a novel by German author Bernard Schlink:

> Often enough in my life I have done things that I had not decided to do. Something . . . goes into action; "it" keeps on smoking although I have decided to quit, and then quits smoking just when I've accepted the fact that I'm a smoker and always will be. I don't mean to say that the thinking and reaching decisions have no influence on behavior. But behavior does not merely enact whatever has already been thought through and decided. It has its own sources.[41]

The Natural History of Addiction

No one is born with addiction. No child wants to be an addict when she grows up. No adolescent starts using a drug with the intention of making a career of addiction. So how does a person despite himself end up with the profound neurological changes of addiction? We have focused on the addicted brain itself; now it is time to put that brain into the context of the chronic disease of addiction. What is the pattern of the addiction? Is it the same for everyone? Is there an alcoholic personality that precedes the development of addiction? Is abstinence necessary to recovery? Can anyone with an addiction safely use her drug of choice in the future? Is treatment helpful?

The answers to these questions are crucial to an understanding of addiction, yet they are hard to come by. Many important observational studies of addiction are an analysis of a cross-section of the population, essentially taking a snapshot of an addicted population at one point in time. Federally funded surveys of American adults' mental health and drug use have interviewed individuals from a large representative sample of households in the United States.[42] Performed annually since 2003, these studies tell us about the prevalence of drug use, the trends among different age groups, but no study informs us about what happens to a single individual over decades. Research studies evaluating the effects of treatment generally follow patients for no more than a few years and often as little as three to six months.

Since addiction is a chronic illness often lasting a lifetime, we must turn to longitudinal studies that have followed the study subjects pro-spectively over many years. It takes a special commitment to do longitudinal research. The researcher must be willing to commit many years of his professional career to this one project; he needs to anticipate what kinds of data will be useful in twenty years and design the study to capture that information. This type of study is expensive, and funding for projects that do not produce short-term results is difficult to secure. As discussed in chapter 1, findings from the longitudinal Minnesota Study of the Development of the Person challenged many assumptions about the antecedents of adolescent drug use.[43] In the second half of the twentieth century, several researchers began to look at what happens over time to a population of people addicted to alcohol.[44] The abuse of alcohol, a common, legal drug, is by far the best studied of the addictions. (While there is a huge amount of research on nicotine as an ingredient in tobacco, I wonder how much interest there would be in nicotine were it not part of the extremely toxic tobacco plant.) Public acceptance of alcohol use and tolerance of alcohol intoxication or abuse give researchers access to a wealth of information about alcohol-related problems. The illicit status of many other addictive drugs distorts our understanding of the natural history of those illnesses and makes it difficult to study the majority of addicted people who are not involved in formal treatment. For example, the opioid addiction of a high-functioning, well-paid businesswoman with the resources to buy her drugs is likely to be invisible to the public eye.

But we should back up. The most informative study is one that follows people prospectively before, during, and after their use of alcohol. Within the field of addiction, there is one such study that has followed two groups of men for seventy-five years. Dr. George Vaillant, a professor of psychiatry at Harvard Medical School and astute observer of the human condition, documents the complex and variable course of alcohol addiction in his two books, *The Natural History of Alcoholism* and *The Natural History of Alcoholism Revisited*,[45] with some reflective thoughts on alcoholism in his 2012 book, *Triumphs of Experience: The Men of the Harvard Grant Study*.[46] His research group followed two cohorts of young white men. The Core City sample included 110 early adolescents from the control group for a study on juvenile delinquency.[47] The College sample of 26 subjects, later expanded to 52, was drawn from a study of Harvard College sophomores selected for their academic prowess and psychological stability. In 1972 these two studies were combined to form the Study of Adult Development directed by Dr. Vaillant.

Both cohorts had extensive initial evaluations of the subjects' physical and social health, habits, and family and social circumstances. Subsequently, subjects were followed with an extensive questionnaire every one to two years and physical examinations every five years. Subjects who did not return questionnaires were interviewed on the telephone or in person every five years. Over a lifetime of follow-up, less than

2 percent of either cohort was lost to the study, a remarkable achievement given the mobility of American society and the effects of chronic alcoholism, such as homelessness and premature death.

We need to understand the results of this longitudinal study in terms of its limitations as well as its strengths. Perhaps the most glaring limitation is the absence of women or people of color as study subjects. We must deal with selection bias, findings skewed because of the population studied, and the racial and gender bias common in the mid-twentieth century. For the purpose of understanding addiction as a disease, a comparison study of different populations might have made this extremely complex subject virtually unfathomable. However, Dr. Vaillant's findings corroborate the findings for the subset of white men in Dr. Dennis Cahalan's national survey of problem drinkers.[48] Other observers before and after Vaillant have had similar findings, suggesting that his work may be more generalizable than one would initially think. Scientific questions and methods have evolved over three decades as knowledge about addictions and about sophisticated scientific methodology has changed. Longitudinal researchers must incorporate new research techniques while maintaining consistency in data collection for the life of the study. Similarly, the terms used for the spectrum of disorders related to drug use have changed with efforts at more accurate definitions. Within the last year, the latest edition of the American Psychiatric Association's *Diagnostic and Statistical Manual of Mental Disorders* (DSM-5) has replaced the discrete categories of "substance abuse" and "substance dependence" with the unitary "substance use disorder," specified as mild, moderate, or severe.[49] This change reflects the thinking in the addictions field that unhealthy substance use and addiction are segments on a continuum. Most importantly, we must remember that the laboratory for this study is the real world. Among the myriad variables that one could study, Dr. Vaillant and his colleagues have chosen variables that seemed most likely to affect the subjects' use of alcohol. However, it is possible that other factors, as yet unknown, will turn out to be more relevant.

Let's look at the findings from Dr. Vaillant's study within the context of alcohol addiction as a chronic illness. Initiation to and heavy use of alcohol as young adults were typical of both cohorts in this study, as in many others.[50] Once subjects' behavior met the criteria for alcoholism,

Vaillant identified two different patterns of longitudinal use: progressive use and atypical use. At age forty-seven, two-thirds of the 110 alcoholic men in the Core City sample manifested a progressive downhill course. One-half of that group were still using alcohol, but the other half had become abstinent. The remaining one-third of men with what Dr. Vaillant calls an "atypical" course of alcoholism were almost evenly split between those who had resumed drinking in an apparently asymptomatic way and those who had developed a homeostasis with their illness. This homeostasis was usually characterized by recurrent remissions and relapses (binges), in spite of which the subjects managed to maintain their jobs and family situations. Thirteen years later, the number of men in each category was fairly constant, but the paths of individual men had varied widely. As an example, eight men who had been drinking heavily at age forty-seven achieved a stable abstinence by age sixty. Conversely, five men with stable abstinence in their midforties had resumed drinking by age sixty.[51] Vaillant contrasts drinking behavior at only a few points in time. The story of one man in the College sample illustrates just how variable the course of this disease may be.

Tom Braceland comments on his alcohol addiction over the course of thirty years. At age twenty-nine, "Alcohol . . . convinces me that the world is better than it seems." Four years later, he muses, "I don't think that I'm an alcoholic, but I drink maybe a quart a week, I am unhappy with less." Within two years, Mr. Braceland seems to control his drinking. "I am changing from a heavy to moderate drinker." Seven years later, at age forty-two, his alcohol addiction is worse: "I drink all day and half the night," forcing him to take more drastic measures. "I quit drinking . . . hopefully for life." At age fifty, he has a relapse, returning to unsafe drinking. His comment "I feel I have alcohol barely under control" becomes a desperate plea by his midfifties. "I really don't want to stop drinking. . . . I hope I can cut down on the booze before it kills me." He appears to attain a more stable remission by age sixty-one. "I am an alcoholic, and I don't drink alcohol. . . . I feel I am beginning to grow."[52]

The nineteen atypical alcoholics in the Core City sample started with the same risk factors as the progressive alcoholism group, but their drinking patterns caused fewer problems with their employment or their marriages. They were likely to binge drink, as much as ten to fifteen drinks daily, but appeared able to manage the timing of their binges to interfere minimally with the rest of their lives. When not bingeing, these atypical alcoholics were usually abstinent and continued to have positive feelings about alcohol. This pattern of recurrent relapses and remission was remarkably stable over thirty to forty years. However, when surveyed at age sixty, these nineteen men had either decreased their drinking or showed signs of progressive disease.[53]

Only a few initial variables could predict significantly[54] whether someone with alcohol addiction would be able to return to asymptomatic, controlled drinking. These men had less severe alcoholism as young adults (fewer problems on the Problem Drinking Scale [PDS] and less out-of-control drinking), fewer alcoholic relatives, and decreased mortality.[55] In contrast to lifelong abstainers in the Core City sample, moderate asymptomatic drinkers were significantly more likely to be married, have better family and social relations, and better physical and mental health.

The College sample men, drawn predominantly from an upper-middle-class background, tended to develop significant problems from alcohol use in the fifth decade, about twenty years later than the Core City sample. Like the Core City atypical alcoholics, the College alcohol abusers generally had a stable pattern of alcohol abuse for twenty to thirty years. The College sample differed in that the occasional periods of out-of-control drinking alternated with heavy drinking, up to ten to fifteen drinks daily, and not with abstinence. These men often appeared as heavy social drinkers, their alcohol-related problems hidden within their families or their own suffering psyches.[56]

There was no evidence of a preexisting alcoholic personality in either of the samples with the exception of those whose behavior had earned them the diagnosis of sociopathy. These individuals were likely to develop severe progressive alcohol dependence in their teens. In his study of deviance in children and adults, Lee Robins reports that adults with childhood histories of deviance had high rates of antisocial behavior, impoverishment, social isolation, and heavy drinking.[57] The question of whether the heavy alcohol use of antisocial people is part of a constellation of social pathologies or is an independent alcohol use disorder has not been settled definitively.

The course of addiction depends on the confluence of variables in the agent (alcohol), the host, and the environment. The changes in brain structure and function induced by heavy drug use lead to behaviors that are frequently beyond the individual's control. Simultaneously, the brain must respond and adapt to alterations in the environment. A major factor in the addicted person's environment is the stigma and discrimination that he faces daily. This stigma extends to his family, to his health care providers, and to his addiction treatment. The prevalence of these negative attitudes about addiction and the impact on addicted people's lives is the subject of the next chapter.

THREE

THE STING OF STIGMA

As a recovering woman, I have personally suffered the scorn of
others who are confused, bitter and misled about addiction. I still
today get the reaction of how could a nice person like me be an
alcoholic. It is hard not to take it personally when I read public
opinion polls of both professionals and the general public who
believe addiction to be a moral weakness rather than a disease.
How could people still believe this in the year 2002?
—First Lady Betty Ford, "Testimony before Join Together
Policy Panel"

Over a decade later, former First Lady Betty Ford's question still reso-
nates.[1] How, indeed? Stigma about addiction reinforces prevailing attitudes. As a social construct, stigma enables dominant groups in society
to define and concentrate their power over groups perceived to be in-
ferior. Usually based on firmly held beliefs, stigma commonly trumps
knowledge of the facts in addressing care and treatment of people with
addiction. This should not surprise us. Beliefs are embedded in powerful
emotions, next to which rationality and intelligence pale. Unfortunately
for a stigmatized group, these opinions of the majority can have devastating consequences. Before looking at these consequences, we need to
understand more about the power of stigma.

The father of French sociology, Emil Durkheim, was one of the first
scholars to think rigorously about stigma. The Dreyfus affair, in which
a Jewish officer in the French army was wrongly convicted of treason,
opened his eyes to the undercurrent of anti-Semitism in French soci-

ety. Durkheim understood Dreyfus's conviction as a way for the French to differentiate the Jewish outsider from mainstream French society.[2] The outsider is perceived as a danger to the social order and morality of the majority. Gerhard J. Falk, professor of sociology at Buffalo State University, elaborates in his book *Stigma: How We Treat Outsiders*: "the stigma and stigmatization of some persons demarcates a boundary that reinforces the conduct of the conformists. Therefore, a collective sense of morality is achieved by the creation of stigma."[3]

Stigma is so pernicious because it allows a social majority to marginalize and devalue another group of human beings under the justification of morality. When stigma is based on an inherent characteristic that a person cannot readily change, such as skin color, gender, or ethnicity, its duplicity and destructive nature is obvious. The last several centuries have given us horrific examples—the enslavement of black Africans by European and American whites, the attempt to eradicate the Jewish people during the Holocaust, the genocide in Rwanda in the 1990s.

Even as the U.S. Constitution provides certain identified groups with protection against discrimination due to race, gender, religion, and national origin, the U.S. Congress has enacted laws that codify discrimination against other groups. When these groups are defined by behaviors perceived as threatening or deviant, the discriminatory nature of stigma may not be as clear. As a society, we punish people whose acts defy our legal code and hurt individuals and their property. Justice demands that people convicted of violent or "white collar" crimes must answer for their behavior. Even after a convicted criminal has paid his dues to society, he is often the lifelong victim of stigmatization that assigns him a primary identity not of his own choosing. No longer a brother, father, or teacher, as the person might describe himself, in society's eyes he is a thief or deviant, first and foremost. As Robin Room, a sociologist who has devoted his career to understanding addiction, points out, "It is also possible to be rich and stigmatized and marginalized, although the affluent are *ipse facto* better able to purchase protection from this."[4] It is not affluence alone that defines this class bias. Stigmatizing someone who has been a prominent member of the dominant society creates an inherent contradiction. We speak of Kenneth Lay as the former chair and chief executive officer of the Enron Corporation who was convicted of fraud, and not primarily as a convicted felon who had served as Enron's chief executive officer.

Then why did Betty Ford, as a member of the powerful elite, come in for such opprobrium? It was because her periods of relapse to alcohol addiction challenged the most basic American ethos of rationalism and self-control. Addiction defies the notion that we freely choose our behaviors on a rational basis. While Ken Lay's behavior was illegal, it was deemed a product of his own values and choices and might not have appeared irrational to some of his peers had he gotten away with it. This idea of the primacy of reason, from the eighteenth-century Age of Enlightenment, was inculcated in the early European settlers. Furthermore, they were an intrepid lot with a strong sense of individual agency. The ability to take care of oneself in this unfamiliar land was important to survival; no wonder individualism and rationality were and still are so highly valued in American society. Any person whose behavior did not conform to the principles of rationality was considered abnormal. And that is still very often what happens. After discussing the case of an addicted patient, my colleague is apt to shake his head, saying, "I still don't understand why anyone would do that to herself." The basic assumption here is that behavior, addictive or not, is freely chosen—an assumption contradicted by more than a decade of solid scientific evidence that addiction is a disease of the brain.

Two American Centuries of Contradictory Ideas about Drugs

We Americans have always held strong beliefs about the use of alcohol, tobacco, and other drugs. Over the past 250 years, our opinions on the matter have fluctuated as customs, politics, public opinion, and the economy have evolved. As a nation, we are ambivalent about any intoxicating substance used primarily for pleasure and enjoyment. The tavern, a respected institution in the late eighteenth century where wealthy landowners could drink and discuss politics and current events, had devolved less than a century later into the saloon, a den of impropriety frequented by miscreants and drunks. Today, drinking alcohol is an accepted, even expected, part of adult social activities for many people, while use of marijuana, a drug with short-term effects similar to alcohol and a better safety profile, is prohibited. Despite knowledge of the health risks of smoking tobacco and the especially addictive nature of nicotine for adolescents, the tobacco industry continues to target the youth market. Drug dealing, legal or illegal, is lucrative business.

How can we understand these contradictory shifting attitudes toward drugs? Access to a particular drug reflects a person's economic status and social environment, prevailing community attitudes regarding drug use, and governmental policy and laws related to the drug. Interestingly, "public" opinion may reflect the passionate views of a vocal minority or the manipulations of those in power and not the desires or behavior of the majority.[5] Prohibition is a good example. While Anti-Saloon League rhetoric provided the vocabulary for discussions of Prohibition, wealthy property owners wanting to ensure a more stable and productive workforce by eliminating access to alcohol were probably more instrumental than the temperance lobby in convincing Congress and state legislatures to pass Prohibition.[6] The public's lack of support, as evidenced by widespread home brewing and the significant market for bootleg alcohol during Prohibition, eventually caused the demise of this ill-advised social policy. Very few Americans alive today would ascribe intoxicated behaviors to supernatural causes, as was common in the seventeenth and eighteenth centuries.[7] But we continue to debate whether addiction and other mental or neurological diseases are illnesses, crimes, or failures of moral character.[8] This contradiction between rhetoric and behavior is a recurrent theme in American drug history.

In the infancy of our republic, all men drank alcohol, and many of them drank all the time. Our forefathers consumed six gallons of distilled spirits per capita annually, three times the current per capita consumption.[9]

The workplace was a social institution and a common arena for drinking. Employers were accepting of the marginal productivity and reliability of their intoxicated workers, until competition became a factor in the marketplace. The consolidation of property by the wealthy and the industrialization of America necessitated a sober and productive workforce. Workshops of skilled craftsmen where men could socialize as they worked gave way to factories employing thousands of low-skilled workers toiling for another's profit. Industrialization ushered in a second era of American attitudes toward drinking: it was antithetical to productive work and subject to abuse no matter what the occasion. These negative attributes formed the backbone of American attitudes about many drugs and alcohol that persist to this day.

Through the mid- and late nineteenth century, the environmental contexts of alcohol and opium use gave both these substances contradictory valences—good as medications, bad as intoxicants. Medicinal laudanum, opium dissolved in alcohol, received wide acceptance in Victorian society, even as smoking opium was decried as dangerous and un-American. Not only was opium dangerous to one's health, but it symbolized the menace of foreigners. A threat from beyond American borders introduced another powerful drug to American society—cocaine from South America. Like the Andean peasants who chewed coca daily to decrease hunger and increase their ability to work at high altitudes, African Americans, destitute and disenfranchised after Reconstruction, likely found that cocaine's stimulating effects could make their lives and work more tolerable. Occasional violent incidents associated with cocaine use assumed mythic proportions and confirmed southern whites' stereotype of African Americans as uncivilized and dangerous. In actuality, whites from all social classes consumed much more cocaine than African Americans. "The exhilarating properties of cocaine made it a favorite ingredient of medicine, soda pop, wines, and . . . a liqueur-like alcohol mixture called Coca Cordial."[10]

By the start of the twentieth century, alcohol, nicotine, opiates, and cocaine were firmly entrenched in American society, although many rural states had outlawed the sale of alcohol as a beverage even as it was making a comeback among the more urban, industrialized populations. Opiates were still widely accepted as medication for many illnesses, while those who used opium for pleasure or escape were denigrated by society. Despite the association of cocaine with violence and destruction, it had found its way into patent medicines and foodstuffs. The formula for the quintessentially American drink Coca-Cola contained 3 percent cocaine until 1903.[11] In keeping with today's antidrug mores, the current

Coca-Cola website contains no mention of cocaine in its history of the famous drink.[12]

As foods or medications containing opium or cocaine came under increased scrutiny, the association of these drugs with marginalized populations—opium and the Chinese; cocaine with South American immigrants and southern African Americans—confirmed their identity as dangerous, foreign substances. Excessive use of tobacco received the same opprobrium as excessive alcohol consumption, but workers recognized that the nicotine in tobacco relieved stress and tension, just as opium, cocaine, and alcohol had made life easier for oppressed Chinese, African Americans, and European immigrant workers.[13] Now, alcohol was destroying America from within; the narcotics from without.

The federal government took advantage of the momentum of the prohibitionist movement to gain control of drug trafficking. State governments had demonstrated a wide range of responses to the threats of the drug trade, many considered lax and unacceptable by the federal government. Using its power to regulate and tax interstate commerce, Congress passed the Harrison Act outlawing the trade of narcotics, except for limited medical and religious purposes. The 1914 law stated that it was unlawful to "produce, import, manufacture, compound, deal in, dispense, sell, distribute or give away" opium and coca products unless the person doing so had registered with the Internal Revenue Service and paid the appropriate tax. The wording of the statute carefully avoided any intimation of restraint of personal liberty. It was legal to use these drugs but, for most people, procuring them was illegal.[14]

Five years later, two Supreme Court cases affirmed the constitutionality of the Harrison Act, including its stipulations requiring physicians to dispense narcotics only by written prescription and as part of professional practice,[15] and prohibiting physicians from prescribing narcotics to treat addiction.[16] Although the Supreme Court based its argument on the issue of federal versus states' rights, this ruling cemented the prevailing attitude that drug addiction was criminal behavior and not a medical issue. This legislation, as interpreted by the 1919 Supreme Court, remains the basis of physicians' prescribing practices for opioids today.

Stigma Closer to Home

Addicted people internalize the social stigma of addiction. Their self-hatred, loss of self-esteem, and shame interfere significantly with their attempts to receive treatment and manage their illness. A patient with opiate addiction reminded me just last month how destructive these internalized feelings could be.

When I first met Bill, he sat in my office berating himself. His primary care physician had referred this twenty-eight-year-old man for a consultation about using Suboxone[17] to manage his heroin addiction. He had started using heroin ten years ago, after his brother died in a car crash when Bill was driving. The drug helped to numb overwhelming feelings of grief and guilt. When he tried to stop heroin, he discovered that he couldn't. Beyond the initial relief, heroin had cost him his job, his savings, and his self-esteem. He had also contracted hepatitis C from sharing needles. And he had only postponed grieving his brother's death. "I am so stupid. I can't do anything right." He sounded angry and disgusted. "And now I have this infection for the rest of my life." His tone of resignation made me wonder if he thought that getting hepatitis C was somehow a just punishment for his heroin addiction. I questioned whether he would even give himself a chance to get well or whether, for an addict, that too was undeserved. My fears were justified; after four weeks, he dropped out of treatment and resumed drug use.

Family members also internalize the stigma accorded the addicted person. They may experience the same shame and self-negation as the addict, even as they are furious about the damage the person's addiction has caused the family. They describe their loved ones stealing repeatedly from family members, lying about it, and becoming enraged when confronted. Driven by the compulsion to use drugs daily, the addicted person needs a substantial, steady cash flow. Unless she has a well-paying job, she has to develop a lifestyle of hustling, cheating, and stealing to pay for drugs. Family cash and household possessions are often the easiest targets. Caught between contradictory impulses to support a loved one or to ostracize her, many families distance themselves from the addicted person for their own self-preservation. The rift between the addict and her family may persist long after the person's addiction is in remission. For the addict trying to recover, her behavior along with the stigma of addiction has cost her a principal form of support at a time when she is most needy and vulnerable to relapse. We know that support from family and friends during a long illness has a demonstrated positive effect on outcome.[18] Certainly an alienated family and a judgmental society, understandable as they are, add up to an environment hostile to recovery from addiction.

Equally important is the role of stigma in shaping the attitudes about addiction of powerful members of the majority culture. When legislators, government officials, or business leaders act on these attitudes, stigma translates into discrimination concretized in laws, policies, employment opportunities, and judicial decisions. This institutionalized discrimination against people with addiction is particularly resistant to change. If a statute is passed that discriminates against people with addiction, one might assume it was based on some hard evidence that justifies the law; therefore, all the negative things about addiction must be true. Sadly, this assumption is often incorrect. In essence, our elected officials have licensed discrimination against people with addiction.

The corporate world has responded to the costs of mental health and addiction problems in the workforce by establishing Employee Assistance Programs (EAP). These programs provide assessment and counseling for psychiatric and addiction issues, among others, usually at an off-site location to ensure the employee's confidentiality. In the year after EAP treatment, employees generate significantly lower health care costs than a comparable group not using EAP resources.[19] But underneath this sensible cost-saving approach to addiction and mental health problems, individual attitudes about addiction still play a cruel role.

Susan Rook knows this all too well. A former host of CNN's *TalkBack Live*, she struggled and succeeded at managing her alcohol and drug addiction with the help and support of CNN. Then, in an upward career move, she landed a plum job with an international communications firm. At a final meeting with her new CEO before starting work, she disclosed that she had had problems with addiction that now had been in remission almost three years. The CEO terminated her on the spot. "How could you ever even begin to think that we would want someone like *you* to represent *us?*"[20]

This CEO expressed the most common attitudes in this country toward addiction. Without even mentioning addiction ("someone like *you*"), this CEO has made it clear that folks with this illness are outliers, not worthy of participating in general society. This CEO is not alone. "Public attitudes toward addiction of any type, but particularly heroin addiction, are overwhelmingly negative. . . . The stereotypes of addicts are of individuals engaged in criminal activity, predatory toward others, and unable or unwilling to respect the norms of acceptable social behavior or participate in the workforce," is the way the Institute of Medicine summarizes public attitudes in its 1995 book on methadone.[21]

The language used to describe addicts and addiction has the power to create its own reality. This linguistic determinism posits that our sense of the world is constructed only in the terms supplied by our language.[22] The popular derogatory language of addiction (junkie, just a drunk, pothead) perpetuates negative attitudes about the illness. For people with minimal understanding of addiction, the current vocabulary of addiction can engender and reinforce stigmatizing beliefs.

Although thoughtful people will avoid derogatory terms like "drunken bum" or "just a junkie," negative attitudes about addiction have infiltrated our language in more subtle ways. Let me illustrate with an example from health care professionals. It is the nature of chronic illnesses to wax and wane in their symptoms. When a person's asthma gets worse, doctors call it an exacerbation. When someone's treated cancer suddenly reemerges, it is a relapse. When a patient's treated addiction suddenly spirals out of control, physicians and nurses call the patient a recidivist— an individual involved in recurrent criminal activity.[23] Language from the criminal justice system subtly supports doctors' and nurses' gut feelings that addiction is more a crime than an illness.

Just as Benjamin Rush, an eighteenth-century American physician, described alcoholism as a disease in 1811,[24] several academic physicians in the 1960s and 1970s decried not only the negative attitudes toward alcoholism of most physicians but also their adverse effects on care for alcohol-dependent patients.[25] Medical education at the time was no help; a study comparing the attitudes of beginning medical students and those of doctors with four to six more years of training found more negative attitudes toward patients with alcoholism as medical training progressed.[26] In the early 1990s, most primary care physicians in a community survey reported having received only a few hours of alcohol/drug education during their training, but very few felt responsible for managing or confident in their management of the disease of alcoholism.[27] A few years later another study of primary care physicians documented that 94 percent felt responsible for advising patients about drinking, but less than a third actually gave any advice.[28] A similar finding in 2009 confirmed that general practitioners (primary care physicians, known as GPs in England) thought that GPs could manage excessive drinking but that there was limited motivation and a lack of perceived competence.[29] Negative attitudes are not limited to physicians. A study of almost three hundred Australian nurses revealed that in response to scenarios of two addicted people admitted to the Emergency Department for complications of drug use, those nurses with more negative affects judged these patients as deserving a lower quality of care.[30] A recent Swedish study found that both mental health professionals and psychiatric patients had similar negative attitudes about people with mental illness.[31]

Given this background, it is not surprising that there is a long history of mutual distrust and often antagonism between physicians and drug-addicted patients admitted to a hospital for other reasons. A small qualitative study of the interactions between hospitalized opioid-addicted patients and their physician teams cataloged four different themes. First, physicians were fearful of being deceived and manipulated by these patients, especially around the issue of prescribing pain medication; second, the physicians did not have any standardized way of assessing these patients, suggesting a lack of training and education in addiction; third, physicians avoided engaging with patients around their concerns for pain meds; and fourth, patients perceived many of their physician's treatment decisions as hostile.[32]

Two quotations from this paper, the first from a patient and the second from a medical doctor in the last year of training, illustrate the problems when doctors have not had adequate training in addiction medicine:

"I mentioned that I would need methadone [*medication to treat opioid withdrawal and severe pain*], and I heard one of them [*physician in training*] chuckle . . . in a negative, condescending way. You're very sensitive because you expect problems getting adequate pain management because you have a history of drug abuse."

". . . since there is this manipulative . . . almost antagonistic interaction, most doctors take the tack of being cautious, and if in error undertreating . . . and in the meantime, the patient is uncomfortable. We just treat them differently."

It's Not Only Stigma; It's Discrimination

In our country, beliefs, including negative attitudes about addiction, are difficult to change, but perhaps our society can begin by addressing discriminatory behaviors. Discrimination, which describes unfair behavior, may be a more useful paradigm than stigma, asserts David Rosenbloom, PhD, the executive director of Join Together, a project at the Boston University School of Public Health, initially funded by the Robert Wood Johnson Foundation and currently part of The Partnership at drugfree.org. Join Together supports community efforts to decrease substance abuse and advocates for fair treatment of addicted people. Dr. Rosenbloom points out that policies or legislation can address discriminatory behaviors that are unfair to people with addiction, but we cannot legislate against stigmatizing beliefs and attitudes.[33] Discrimination is a term the American people understand, he continues, because it speaks to a basic sense of justice and fairness. If American people perceive the negative treatment of addicted people as a form of discrimination, they may support addicts' rights not to be victims of discrimination despite their belief that addicts choose their negative behaviors willfully. The rest of this chapter examines the effects of discriminatory statutes and policies on people with addiction. The primary focus will be on barriers to receiving appropriate treatment for addiction, including the context in which people must live with this illness.

Addiction treatment in the United States reflects the prevailing erroneous paradigm of addiction as an acute illness. A serious acute illness requires intensive treatment initially followed by a period of monitoring until the person is cured. An addicted person actively using drugs gets care first at a detoxification center, where the primary purpose is to help the person get the drug out of his system safely. Depending on the person's resources, the next step may be an intensive inpatient or outpatient rehabilitation program for one to four weeks, followed by weekly counseling or group therapy for several months, or no treatment at all. Medications may be given for just a few months. The addicted person has then "completed" treatment, and any return to drug use represents a personal failure. Physicians more often than not will state that a person has failed treatment, rather than the treatment failed to stem the disease. Conspicuously absent from this paradigm is the continuity of health care that enables people to manage ongoing chronic health problems.

In contrast, let's look at the treatment of cardiovascular disease. A heart attack certainly requires acute hospital intervention and care. The patient leaves the hospital on several medications with the expectation he may need them for the rest of his life to decrease his risk of further heart attacks. He may receive some cardiac rehabilitation for several weeks or months. Once out of the hospital, he returns to his community physician for management of his cardiac disease, perhaps with the help of a consulting cardiologist. The patient and his doctor assume that he will need ongoing monitoring of his heart problems with significant attention to making changes in his lifestyle—his diet, exercise regime, and management of stress. The goal is to retard the progression of the illness and prevent another heart attack. Should he have another heart attack, a relapse if you will, he receives more intensive treatment and the sympathy of friends and family—a stark contrast to the opprobrium an addicted person receives when his illness recurs. If we were to apply this chronic disease model to addiction, primary care providers (physicians, physician assistants, advanced practice nurses) would need to have the skills to monitor their addicted patients, manage medications, and work on relapse prevention. More specialized addiction treatment would need to be readily available for those patients needing intensive care.

Addiction treatment in the United States is many years away from this model of chronic disease management. "The current treatment system is a barrier to (addicted) people getting well," was Dr. Rosenbloom's succinct assessment. He quickly pointed out that his comment was not a condemnation of those working in the addictions field, many of whom care for the sickest addicted people with commitment and compassion despite paltry resources. The field of addiction both in research and in service delivery is chronically underfunded. The number of available services is inadequate, and those that exist are not all of high quality.[34] The lack of training in addiction for doctors, nurses, and other health care professionals serves as a major impediment to improved care.[35] Without adequate knowledge about addiction, health care personnel discriminate against addicted people in ways that may compromise the addicted person's care for all his health problems.[36]

How did we get into this mess? A look at the evolution of care for people with addictions suggests some answers. In the nineteenth and early twentieth centuries, the impetus to protect society from the annoyance or corrupting influence of addicted people and behaviors such as public drunkenness led to the development of traditions and institutions aimed to remove the addict from public view. Until the middle of the twentieth century, many cities had laws against public drunkenness, even without disruptive behavior. The policy of protective custody allowed police departments to hold intoxicated people overnight, ostensibly for their own good. Inebriated people were arrested and jailed until they sobered up, a potentially life-threatening situation for those at risk for the most serious alcohol withdrawal syndrome, delirium tremens.

A more modern example is the structure and oversight of methadone maintenance treatment (MMT) programs today. In a study of women in MMT, Jennifer Friedman documents the intensive surveillance these women experience. They report giving urine specimens for drug testing under direct observation of program staff and having their methadone dosage arbitrarily decreased or terminated as "punishment" for having evidence of other drug use in urine specimens.[37] Imagine taking away a diabetic person's medication because she had eaten a piece of cake! Both these patients need more help controlling their illnesses, not less.

These women experienced the process of methadone maintenance as "demeaning and abusive." Professor Friedman argues that methadone clinics are a disciplinary institution to teach women to monitor themselves — not a medical treatment. On methadone, these women are "safe deviants."

They subject themselves to the power dynamic and values of the dominant society in exchange for a needed medication.[38]

While methadone controls an addicted person's craving for heroin, it cannot change the patterns of manipulative and devious behavior developed over years of addiction. Learning new more appropriate behaviors takes time and practice. We should expect that some clients in MMT will exhibit the antisocial behaviors they developed as part of their illness, but to base a program on the assumption that all clients will behave in this way reinforces the paradigm that drug-addicted people are outsiders not entitled to respect or trust. Unfortunately, these attitudes can have fatal consequences.

Jackie liked the pain medication Percocet, a combination of the semisynthetic opioid oxycodone and acetaminophen, and when her addiction was active, she liked it better than anything else. At her first visit to me, her new primary care doctor, the telltale signs of a drug problem were there: pain syndromes without objective pathology (migraine headaches and pelvic pain), several medications with addictive potential, a vague history about her prior physicians, no old medical records, and an insistent request for some Percocet for her really bad headaches. We got to know each other very well over the next fifteen years. Born into a large Irish family, she had grown up with family alcoholism and the attendant abuse and chaos. She was tough, scrappy, and generous. For years, she coached a girls' softball team and with her husband put on an annual Valentine's Day charity event. And she struggled with addiction, Percocet if she could get it, several thousand dollars of scratch tickets a week when she wasn't using drugs, and always nicotine. Even after the loss of a leg from severe circulation problems due in part to her smoking, she was unable to quit. She had one or two relapses to Percocet yearly: she would be edgy and irritable at our visits; then she would stop showing up. Eventually I would get a call from a detoxification or addiction rehabilitation program telling me that she was being discharged. Jackie worked very hard to keep her addiction in remission. She attended several Alcoholics Anonymous (AA) meetings a week, speaking to her AA sponsor daily; she worked with her therapist weekly. She even asked her mother or her husband to hold on to her medications and to manage her paycheck so that she would not be tempted to abuse her medications or spend her cash on drugs.

When she decided to go on methadone, her life changed. Without the craving, she was no longer frenetic. She was able to take care of the increasing number of addiction-related health problems: pneumonia, acute kidney failure, loss of circulation in her legs. The methadone to treat her addiction offered the additional benefit of treating her chronic leg pain.

One day she saw another MMT client whom she barely knew walking toward the methadone clinic. Jackie stopped and offered her a ride. While Jackie went in to get her medication, this woman tried to sell drugs out of Jackie's car. For her acquaintance's infraction, Jackie was terminated from the methadone program. She was desperate and afraid. Once her methadone was tapered and discontinued, she had at least a four-week wait to get into another program. We talked about how she might keep herself safe from relapse—more meetings, more counseling, more contact with her sponsor. It wasn't enough. A few days later I got a call from an Emergency Department physician: Jackie had been brought in by the emergency medical technicians not breathing, and the trauma team could not revive her. The only drug found in her blood was methadone. Presumably, she bought some methadone on the street—maybe her usual dose. But, now that her body was not tolerant to the sedative effects of methadone, it was enough to kill her.[39]

Jackie's death was unnecessary. Did she make bad decisions? Yes. Should she have been more careful about the people with whom she hung out? Undoubtedly. The staff members at her MMT program had their side of the story; I had heard only Jackie's. The action taken by her MMT program, one of the best in our area, typifies both the standard of care and the punitive approach at many MMT programs. But I can think of no other illness in which behavior indicating the need for more treatment would be addressed by denying essential treatment.

Since nineteenth- and twentieth-century society understood addiction as a criminal and moral issue, there was no impetus for physicians to be involved or even interested. The only known medical treatment for addiction—prescribing opiates for persons with morphine or opium addiction—had been a federal crime since the passage of the Harrison Act in 1914. Many physicians in the twentieth century did not consider addressing a patient's habits within the purview of the medical profession.

In the absence of scientific interest in addiction, Alcoholics Anonymous (AA), a lay organization dedicated to helping people stop drinking, became the source of information about alcoholism for the public and for health care professionals. While many of AA's precepts for managing alcohol addiction demonstrate impressive psychological insight and sophistication, AA dogma explaining the disease of alcoholism has led to inaccurate perceptions of addiction by the general public. According to AA, alcoholism always has a progressive downhill course until the person dies or recovers; each person's addiction has an immutable path and cannot be changed until she reaches a nadir, her "rock bottom"; and a person is powerless over her addiction and must turn to a spiritual "higher power" to recover. I want to emphasize that many members of AA have a more sophisticated understanding of their disease based on scientific evidence. But the message that addiction is a hopeless condition, against which a person is helpless without the occurrence of an inexplicable, almost miraculous, turnaround, has permeated the public imagination for three-quarters of a century.

Treatment and Social Control

Given this widespread defeatist perception of addiction, it should not surprise us that current addiction treatment is inadequate in many areas: availability of treatment, quality of programs and staff, access to treatment, and access to ongoing support. Let's start with an addicted person's access to care and treatment. Over a twelve-month period, only 12 percent of people with alcoholism receive any medical or lay (AA and other mutual help groups) treatment for their illness, while over a lifetime, only one-quarter will have some contact with any kind of treatment.[40] Only a fraction of those people receive care from addiction specialists. The majority are seen in primary care or emergency settings, where their illness goes unnoticed most of the time. Even when it is recognized, physicians refer only a small fraction of their addicted patients for care and manage even fewer. These numbers have remained stable over the last two to three decades, despite increased public awareness of alcohol and drug problems.[41]

What happens to the more than 85 percent of addicted people who are essentially on their own? In his longitudinal study of alcoholism, Dr. George Vaillant found that those whose alcoholism was in remission credited their recovery to a new stable intimate relationship, a healthier "addiction" (exercise or attending AA meetings), or a severe medical complication related to drinking.[42] There are many ways to recover without formal medical help. Vaillant notes that approximately one-third of people with alcoholism do have a severe progressive downward course, but the other two-thirds either become abstinent or develop a homeostasis with their drinking (a lot of alcohol but few major adverse complications). This number compares similarly, and even favorably, with the prognoses for other chronic diseases: only half of American adults with chronic hypertension have their blood pressure controlled,[43] and over one-quarter of people with diabetes are unaware of their disease and are not receiving treatment.[44] When I look at the estimates of how many people with hypertension, diabetes, or addiction have their illnesses well controlled, I am struck by how similar the figures are. Taking care of such chronic illnesses is hard work for everyone.

Chronic diseases are a major economic burden on our society, both in terms of the lost productivity of disabled people unable to work and in terms of health care costs. In 2010 the United States spent $44 billion to treat diabetes, which affects 26 million people; $87 billion to treat cancer, which affects 19 million people; and $107 billion to treat heart conditions, which affect 27 million people. In contrast, the United States spent only $28 billion to treat the 40 million people with addiction.[45]

The amounts of public funding through the National Institutes of Health for treatment and research on addiction and other chronic illnesses highlight the low priority for addiction. What makes these figures particularly striking is that the top five leading causes of morbidity and mortality in this country (heart disease, cancer, chronic lower respiratory diseases, stroke, and accidents), which account for 63 percent of all deaths,[46] are caused or exacerbated by alcohol and drug use and addiction. The National Institute on Drug Abuse (NIDA) and the National Institute on Alcohol Abuse and Alcoholism (NIAAA) had a combined budget of $1.5 billion in 2012. The National Heart Lung Blood Institute budget is twice this size, while the National Cancer Institute has a budget three times NIDA's and NIAAA's combined budgets.[47] Not only are there too few specialized addiction programs, but the quality is often in question. Certainly, money and good health insurance can buy excellent care. There are nationally known programs such as the Betty Ford Center at Rancho Mirage, California, and Hazelden in Minnesota, where a four-week residential program costs about $20,000 to $30,000.[48] Few people have the resources to access these programs. Inadequate public funding for addiction treatment programs can compromise their quality. A 2002 study of methadone maintenance programs found that only one-third of the programs were providing recommended doses of methadone, despite having received a Treatment Improvement Protocol for MMT programs published in 1996 by NIDA and the Substance Abuse and Mental Health Services Administration (SAMHSA) and mailed to all nationally listed MMT programs.[49] Poorly resourced programs serving African Americans or those programs favoring a detoxification model of treatment used even lower doses.

An inadequately trained workforce presents another significant barrier to high-quality treatment. The medical profession has abdicated responsibility for ensuring that medical students and doctors in training receive adequate teaching in addiction disorders. Despite the high prevalence of addictive disorders, most medical schools offer between three and twelve hours of addictions curriculum over four years.[50] Nursing, social work, and dental students fare worse.[51] On the postgraduate level, addiction training is even more scattered. Resident physicians learn about managing the serious medical complications of addiction — infections of the heart valves, pneumonia, and severe trauma — but not about the disease of addiction itself. The 1990 report from the Institute of Medicine, *Broadening the Base of Treatment for Alcohol Problems*, recommended that prevention, identification, and treatment of alcohol problems occur in community health and primary care settings.[52] That report has fallen on deaf ears. In general, medical centers have ignored recommendations to shift care for alcohol-related problems into community settings in order to identify and intervene earlier in alcohol problems and continue to monitor people in their own communities. At the same time, primary care physicians who are managing patients with other common chronic diseases—diabetes, heart disease, hypertension, emphysema, osteoarthritis—shy away from "those patients" with addiction. Over the past thirty years, there have been increasing efforts to educate practicing clinicians, students, and faculty in various health professions about substance use and abuse. The Association for Medical Education and Research in Substance Abuse (AMERSA), in collaboration with the Bureau of Health Professions, Health Resources and Services Administration (HRSA) and SAMHSA, developed a national blueprint for interdisciplinary substance abuse education for health professionals. During seven years of funding, Project Mainstream trained over ten thousand health professionals in more than twelve disciplines at twenty different health professions' institutions.[53] This was a massive undertaking, but only the very beginning of what's needed. In a 2012 report, *Addiction Medicine: Closing the Gap between Science and Practice,* researchers at the National Center on Addiction and Substance Abuse at Columbia University (CASA-Columbia) concluded that "medical professionals . . . receive little education or training in addiction science, prevention and treatment." Further, "addiction counselors, who make up the largest share of providers of addiction treatment services, provide care for patients with a medical disease yet they are not required to have any medical training and most states do not require them to have advanced education of any sort."[54] The essential missing ingredient in all these efforts is the persistent political will in universities, medical centers, and state and federal governments to promulgate evidence-based programs—clinical and educational—to treat people with addictions.

Parity? Not Yet

In most illnesses, the patient and her doctor decide together on the type and length of treatment. The clinician makes treatment recommendations based on research evidence, clinical experience, and the patient's preferences. Two patients with hypertension may choose different, but equally effective, medications because of differences in side effects and lifestyle. In addiction treatment, insurance companies and established treatment protocols rather than the team of patient and physician make these decisions. With limited resources for addiction treatment, physicians have little opportunity to individualize their patients' addiction care. Insurance companies have argued that providing unlimited coverage for addiction and other mental health problems would be prohibitively expensive for their companies, but research indicates that insurance payments would rise no more than a few dollars annually per enrollee.[55]

For many years, health insurance companies were able to limit the type and amount of substance abuse treatment. If the chronic illness had been heart disease or asthma, no one would have tolerated these restrictions. The 2008 Mental Health and Addiction Equity Act addressed the parity issue for the approximately 45 percent of American residents who get their health insurance through large employer groups or state-regulated plans (100 million) and Medicaid-managed care plans (39 million). In full effect since 2011, this law requires that those insurers already providing mental health and substance use disorder benefits must provide them in a "no more restrictive" manner than the provision of medical and surgical benefits.[56] As of 2014, in compliance with the mandates of the Patient Protection and Affordable Care Act of 2010,[57] all insurance plans participating in state health insurance exchanges and Medicaid must cover mental health and substance abuse services that comply with the parity act. These laws have the potential to improve access to addiction care significantly, but a recent study of access to such care in Massachusetts following the implementation of that state's universal health care law is a cautionary tale.[58] The authors conclude: "Among other factors, our study noted that the percentage of uninsured patients with substance abuse issues remains relatively high—and that when patients did become insured, requirements for copayments on their care deterred treatment. Our analysis suggests that expanded coverage alone is insufficient to increase treatment use. Changes in eligibility, services, financing, system design, and policy may also be required."

In a sobering 2013 report on three studies funded by the American Society of Addiction Medicine, researchers found that both Medicaid and commercial health insurance plans limit access to medications for opiate addiction, despite robust evidence of medical efficacy and cost-effectiveness.[59] Insurers impose quantity and dosage limits and requirements for prior authorizations for these medications to a much greater degree than for medications for other chronic diseases. Adequate coverage for appropriate psychosocial treatments is also hard to come by. Is this parity? My patient HM wouldn't think so.

HM, a forty-two-year-old mail carrier, is sitting anxiously in my office. Over the last several years, he used alcohol to deal with increasing memories and fears related to childhood trauma. Recently, he realized that he could not stop drinking and sought help from his union. After a four-day hospital detoxification, his union's health insurer agreed to cover only outpatient treatment, although the patient, struggling with both alcohol addiction and post-traumatic stress disorder (PTSD), had requested more intensive residential treatment to prevent relapse. When he relapsed within a few days, his union found him a thirty-day residential treatment program. However, his insurance agreed to cover only one week of treatment. When I called his insurance company to protest, nonmedical personnel told me that longer residential treatment was "not medically necessary." HM has since relapsed again, required another detoxification, and is trying to cobble together an outpatient program that his insurance will cover.

These existing gatekeeper controls make it more difficult for an addicted population already reluctant to get care to receive needed treatment. And what is the situation for those whose health insurance plans are not regulated by the Affordable Health Care Act of 2010? Smaller businesses with fewer than fifty-one employees are exempt, and others operate in states that do not require health insurance companies to provide any mental health or addiction benefits. Insurance companies have cut costs by offering the fewest benefits allowed under states' laws. Like HM's insurance company, many private insurers have decided that outpatient addiction treatment is more effective than inpatient care. Certainly the price is better. Fortunately research confirms that many people will do well with outpatient care, but there are some people who will need more intensive inpatient care that their insurance companies may not cover.

The important point here is that for people with addiction, clinical decisions are not made within the context of a clinician-patient relationship but by insurance company executives more committed to the health of their profits than the health of those insured.

Adequate enforcement of these laws will be an ongoing problem because of their complexity and lack of specific standards.[60] Monitoring managed care organizations, each with several different plans, would confound even a well-funded and organized insurance enforcement effort; so it is no surprise that most states are unable to monitor and enforce insurance statutes adequately. Furthermore, advocacy groups composed of health care providers often think their work is done once a bill is passed, whereas ongoing monitoring is required to ensure implementation of the new laws. This is the assessment of Deb Beck, a social worker, tenacious lobbyist, and advocate for addicted people. Deb started out as a counselor caring for the most down-and-out people with alcoholism in Harrisburg, Pennsylvania. Frustrated by the lack of public resources for her patients, she moved into the political arena as a consultant and lobbyist on the state and national levels. When she learned that in Pennsylvania there were "lobbyist(s) for parking meters, Ferris wheels, and jukeboxes, but none for people with alcohol and drug problems," her career course was set.[61]

Meanwhile, there is another statute that interferes with good medical care and protects the insurance companies' bottom lines. The Uniform Accident and Sickness Policy Provision law (UPPL), promulgated as a model law by the National Association of (state) Insurance Commissioners (NAIC) in 1947 and adopted by more than three-quarters of state legislatures, allows a health insurer to deny coverage if an insured person with acute trauma has any documented evidence of alcohol intoxication or unprescribed narcotic use on admission to a medical facility. If so, the hospital is unlikely to get paid, and the patient may be saddled with significant medical debt, which happens to be the major cause of personal bankruptcy in the United States.[62] Physicians may therefore be reluctant to document a patient's blood alcohol concentration, despite evidence that addressing the person's intoxication (with or without addiction) leads to improved health outcomes.[63] Thirty-five states still have this provision on their books, although the NAIC, the originator of UPPL, has recommended its repeal since 2001.

Discrimination against Addicted People Blights Other Aspects of Their Lives

Many chronic illnesses are disabling; addiction is no exception. However, federal regulations state that addiction, no matter how severe, does not qualify as a disability, although severe medical complications of addiction may qualify. No person is eligible for Social Security Disability Insurance benefits solely on the basis of her addiction, whereas medical complications such as morbid obesity, possibly rooted in a compulsive eating disorder, or chronic lung disease from a lifetime of smoking, do meet these criteria for disability.[64] Trying to manage an addiction without any income is difficult enough, but former Senator Phil Gramm (R-Texas) wanted to make clear that addicted people do not deserve any public entitlements. His amendment to the Welfare to Work Act of 1996 prohibits anyone convicted of a drug felony from *ever* receiving public housing, public welfare, or food stamps. This legislation imposes a lifetime sentence on even nonviolent drug offenders convicted of possession or selling of controlled substances.[65] Violent offenders convicted of non-drug-related crimes are not subject to such punitive measures. Young adults convicted of a drug felony are also barred from receiving future federal education loans if convicted while using a student loan.[66] Addicted people are right, concludes David Rosenbloom. "Society is out to get them."

While these facts are an indictment of our society, the solutions are clear. The U.S. Preventive Services Task Force has named substance abuse as one of its top health priorities for the Healthy People 2020 program.[67] Join Together, in its report "Ending Discrimination," outlines ten recommendations for addressing discrimination against people with addictions in health care, employment, and public benefits (table 3.1).[68]

These recommendations are a useful tool, but only if interested members of the community stand up and take action. "We need to educate our elected officials," Deb Beck urges, to understand that addiction is a brain disease and recognize the discriminatory nature of statutes and

Table 3.1 Join Together's Ten Recommendations to End Discrimination in Health Care

Health care	1. Insurance coverage for treatment of substance use disorders (SUD) should be at parity with that for other illnesses. 2. Insurers should not be allowed to deny claims for the care of any injury sustained by an insured person if he or she was under the influence of alcohol or other drugs at the time of injury. 3. Treatment for SUD should be personalized to each patient, and based on the best scientific protocols and standards of care, including the use of appropriate medications, behavioral therapies, and ancillary services.
Employment	4. Employees who voluntarily seek treatment for SUD should not be subject to discriminatory actions or dismissal. 5. Past alcohol or other drug use should be considered only when relevant to the job.
Public benefits	6. People with drug convictions but no current drug use should face no obstacles getting student loans, other grants, scholarships, or access to government training programs. 7. Persons with nonviolent drug convictions but no current drug use should not be subject to bans on receiving cash assistance and food stamps. 8. Public housing agencies and providers of Section 8 and other federally assisted housing should use the discretion given to them in the public housing law to help people get treatment, rather than permanently barring them and their families from housing. 9. People who are disabled as a result of their SUD should be eligible for Social Security Disability Income and Supplemental Security Income. 10. Decisions involving the custodial status of children should be made in the best interests of a child based on what is happening in the home.

Source: Adapted from Join Together Policy Panel (2003).

policies. NIDA and NIAAA need the freedom to publicize the findings of their funded research, rather than the political agenda of whatever administration is in the White House. We deserve a health care workforce with the knowledge and skills to treat addictions and a health care system committed to high-quality care to address the illness that affects one in four American families.[69]

FOUR

RISK AND RESILIENCE

One child in an apparently well-adjusted middle-class family develops alcohol addiction, while her siblings have successful careers and healthy families. One child growing up in economic and social deprivation seems impervious to the negative influences around him as his parents and siblings succumb to addiction. These vignettes highlight the individualized nature of people's responses to circumstance. The more we understand about these individuals, the less idiosyncratic their successes or tragedies seem. Common themes emerge about individual vulnerabilities and strengths, as well as environmental risks and resources.

Human resilience and vulnerability come into play only in the context of an adverse experience such as addiction. When a person's life is going well, there is no need of resilience, and vulnerability to certain stresses may not be tested. Resilience and vulnerability are developmental processes, not static characteristics. Both represent learned cognitive, emotional, and behavioral responses to stimuli whether internal and genetically influenced or external environmental conditions. While we would likely all agree that resilience is a positive process, this chapter will present evidence that vulnerability is not necessarily wholly negative. Vulnerability and resilience develop in response to specific experiences; many factors influence whether these responses become more generalized. Most commonly, resilience and vulnerability to different circumstances exist in a unique combination in each person, often making it difficult to predict how someone will respond to challenging situations, such as relapse to addictive behaviors.

Resilience is the process of learning how to cope successfully despite negative experiences. It requires attributes and skills that differ at each level of development. In response to the death of a beloved grandparent, a young girl may just want to go play with her friends, while her grieving mother rationalizes her loss as God's will. Some forms of resilience seem innate to the organism. A child may recover quickly from a viral illness, while her parents feel tired and achy for days. Some attributes are shaped by the environment, such as the self-confidence of a child raised in a warm and supportive family. Other aspects of resilience are acquired, often intentionally, such as the cognitive and emotional maturity that allows most adults to function effectively and independently in the world. Professor Michael Rutter, a British psychiatrist who has studied resilience for many years, puts it this way: "Resilience is an interactive concept that is concerned with the combination of serious risk experiences and a relatively positive psychological outcome despite those experiences. . . . it implies a relative resistance to environmental risk experiences, or the overcoming of stress or adversity."[1]

Vulnerability, an increased susceptibility to the negative effects of a challenging experience, represents the opposite end of the continuum. Like resilience, vulnerability also represents a process and interaction between genetically programmed innate characteristics and an individual's responses to the environment. The wide variety of responses to a particular negative event demonstrates that each of us will respond with a unique combination of resilience and vulnerability based on our innate characteristics, prior experiences, and current circumstances.

After the World Trade Center attacks of September 11, 2001, my most resilient patients were those with histories of emotional trauma who already understood that the world was an unsafe place and had learned how to survive and manage their lives in such an ambiguous state of being. Patients who had lived a life of presumed American invulnerability were deeply shaken. And for my patients actively struggling with overwhelming mental health or addiction problems, the tragic events of 9/11 only confirmed their fears of how dangerous and unsafe their own lives were.

The complex interactions of individual genetic and environmental factors will influence whether an individual might succumb to the pressures of adversity or manage to cope, but our understanding of these factors does not allow us to predict with certainty the outcome following any particular adverse event. This assumption of unpredictability seems a matter of quantity of variables rather than a qualitative distinction between measurable and immeasurable forces. Were we able to catalog instantaneously the billions of interactions from the molecular and cellular level to macro forces in the environment, we might find that all outcomes are the products of physical, chemical, and biological laws and matter. Such a deterministic assertion seems more palatable when applied to an overwhelming genetic or environmental factor, such as profound mental retardation or a childhood of physical and emotional abuse. Despite exciting leaps in the understanding of genetics and the expression of genetic material in the object world, our understanding of what enables resilience or vulnerability is still rudimentary.

Addiction Forges Strength; It Also Kills

To make sense of this extremely complex field of risk and response as it applies to addiction, it may be helpful to approach it from three different perspectives. The first is to appreciate the fluidity of the development of resilience and vulnerability. We are looking at the complex human organism as it grows from infant to adult through many developmental stages, each dependent on the prior stages and current environment.[2] Addiction itself takes years to develop, beginning with learned cultural behaviors around use of drugs and continuing through repeated assaults on the brain's basic reward pathways to the uncontrollable use of a drug. Research data have given us many snapshots of gene-environment interactions, but for now, to appreciate the accretion of vulnerability and resilience over time, literature may guide our understanding better than science.

A central conflict in Shakespeare's *Hamlet*[3] is Hamlet's inability to act as his father's son and "Revenge his foul and most unnatural murther" (act I, scene v). This genetic imperative drives Hamlet's self-hatred to the brink of suicide to escape his own thoughts: "I could be bounded in a nutshell and count myself a king of infinite space, were it not that I have bad dreams" (act II, scene ii) and the environment's "slings and arrows of outrageous fortune" (act III, scene i). In capturing the intricate inter-weaving of genetic and environmental factors, Shakespeare articulates the philosophy that while we cannot control the genetic and environ-mental factors that forge our lives, neither are we pawns to those forces. We have a glimpse perhaps of Shakespeare's understanding of resilience in Hamlet's words "the readiness is all" (act V, scene ii). Hamlet cannot predict his future, but he can bring his skills, experience, and determi-nation to the challenge of avenging his father's murder.

The second perspective acknowledges that ever-changing external en-vironmental pressures and internal thoughts and feelings produce mil-lions of gene-environment interactions. When attempting to trace their results, where do we draw the boundary between internal and external? A cell biologist might consider everything outside the cell membrane to be the environment; the geneticist would rightly say that everything out-side the genome is environment. At the other end of the scale, a family or community could be the unit of study for social scientists. Because we are investigating the disease of addiction in humans, it makes sense for the person to be our unit of study, but we need to realize that the choice is arbitrary. Studying the effects of gene-environment interactions on human behavior is a broad endeavor, encompassing many scientific dis-ciplines with different paradigms. Extrapolating these diverse findings to the realm of human behavior requires attention to these differences. Our discussion will draw on qualitative and quantitative data from the natural and social sciences, psychology, and clinical medicine.

The third perspective requires a step back from specific gene-environment interactions and the limits of current scientific technique. Broad social, political, and cultural forces determine the choice of re-search endeavors via funding priorities and the interpretation of results. Large secular trends such as American attitudes about alcohol and drugs will affect their availability and the consequences of using them. Ideas about the role of children in society as students, as workers, as responsi-ble adults have created opportunities for the development of addiction. We might speculate, for instance, that the prolonged adolescence of privileged American children as they complete their secondary school, college, and postgraduate education, often without significant responsi-bilities to or for others, provides fertile ground for experimentation with and possible addiction to drugs. Differing sociopolitical views on our obligation as a society to support the welfare of the most disadvantaged among us clearly affects the choices and opportunities of marginalized groups. Children who grow up in poverty, and/or who start using drugs as young adolescents, and/or who drop out of school without marketable skills are more vulnerable to the allure of drugs. A dearth of positive environmental stimulation and an inability to effect changes in their own lives create a situation ripe for addiction. Animal research data confirm that laboratory rats housed in a nonstimulating environment use drugs because they provide the only significant reward in that environment.[4]

An exhaustive review of environmental and genetic factors influencing resilience and vulnerability across the span of human development and addiction would rightly require an entire book. The discussion here is intended to be illustrative rather than exhaustive. As we examine the evidence through each lens, I shall endeavor to describe categories of effects and interactions, providing examples from different scientific disciplines.

The Development of the Person

Two themes emerge in tracing the development of the person: early effects may have consequences much later in life, and the toxicity of early events may often be attributed to the immaturity of the organism's development. Let us look at five stages of human development: fetal growth, infancy, early childhood, adolescence, and adulthood.

The rapid development of a fetus from a single cell to an infant in just nine months makes it particularly vulnerable to the environmental effects of drugs. Most drugs, prescribed or illicit, taken by a pregnant woman do cross the placenta into the bloodstream of the fetus. Women addicted to nicotine who continue to smoke during pregnancy have babies with lower birth weights.[5] Heavy doses of alcohol ingested by a pregnant woman may produce offspring with mental retardation, emotional and behavioral difficulties, and, in the extreme, characteristic changes in facial features (fig. 4.1).[6] This constellation of deleterious effects, known as fetal alcohol spectrum disorder, is one of the leading causes of mental retardation in the United States.[7] Pregnant women who are able to stop

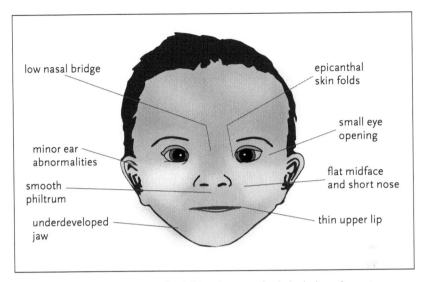

low nasal bridge

epicanthal
skin folds

small eye
opening

minor ear
abnormalities

flat midface
and short nose

smooth
philtrum

underdeveloped
jaw

thin upper lip

Fig. 4.1 Typical facial features of a child with severe fetal alcohol syndrome.
Adapted from Warren, Hewitt, and Thomas (2011), courtesy of National Institute
on Alcohol Abuse and Alcoholism.

drinking during pregnancy are likely to have healthier children.[8] Newborn infants continue to be susceptible to the toxic effects of drugs and
of common medications, as their livers are not sufficiently developed to
metabolize them.

In infancy, the attachment between an infant and caregiver plays a
crucial role in a child's development.[9] This primary relationship, involving powerful, unarticulated emotions, underlies a child's later sense of
self-worth. The licking and grooming behavior of a mother rat during
her pup's first week of life changes the growing pup's response to stress
by inducing alterations in the pup's gene expression.[10] Human nurturing
behavior may have a similar effect.

Childhood, usually free from the direct toxic effects of drugs, is a time
for development of generic strengths and vulnerabilities. Good parenting skills and a positive parent-child relationship are closely related to
positive childhood development. A warm and trusting relationship leads
to competence and positive self-esteem, both important components of
resilience. Conversely, maternal depression and a lack of positive mother-
child interactions can have a negative impact on development.[11] Addi-

tional adverse early childhood experiences create a cumulative risk for poor behavioral outcomes in later childhood and adolescence.[12] And, for better or worse, prior behavior exerts a conforming pressure on current behavior.[13] We shall examine further the data supporting these generalizations in the discussion of external environmental influences on vulnerability and resilience.

Adolescence brings new developmental concerns. We know that experimentation and use of drugs generally starts in adolescence—when the brain areas responsible for judgment, prioritizing, and executive decision making are not fully formed—and lasts until the brain reaches maturity in the midtwenties. The brains of adolescent rats respond to nicotine, alcohol, and cocaine in ways that lead to increased susceptibility to heavy use and addiction as adult rats. Observations from scientists and tobacco company marketers confirm many of these behaviors in human teens.[14] On a drug-specific level, adolescents who require higher doses of alcohol to experience its intoxicating effects have a significantly increased risk of alcohol dependence as adults.[15] While drug use can damage some of the developing neurotransmitter systems, such as dopamine and gamma-aminobutyric acid,[16] it is unlikely that drug use alone explains addiction problems that develop in adulthood. Many other genetic and environmental factors contribute to the brain's vulnerability.

The sharp decline in incidence of addiction after the age of twenty-five suggests that physiologic maturity is in itself protective. But, as William Wordsworth said with eloquent simplicity, "The child is father to the man."[17] Childhood experiences may provide manageable challenges that, when mastered, enhance one's opportunities to succeed at all stages of development, leading to competence and flexibility. Unfortunately, the converse is also true. For adults with persistent addictive behavior, a combination of genetic and environmental factors may perpetuate their addictions. Variations in genetic coding for dopamine correlate with the degree of impulsive behavior. People with high impulsivity and propensity for risk taking have increased vulnerabilities to addiction.[18] Genetic susceptibilities to depression, sociopathy, or other forms of major mental illness will increase vulnerability to addiction. That over two-thirds of people with an addictive disorder also suffer from a major mental illness should not be surprising given the common neurological systems involved.[19]

The interplay of four sets of factors—general environmental, personal, addiction-related, and drug-specific—contributes to the development of addiction. While exposure to an addictive substance is necessary for drug addiction, the substance alone is never sufficient explanation for the development of addiction. Many physicians and patients alike do not understand this basic concept. Doctors hesitate to prescribe pain medications with addictive properties, and many patients are fearful of taking needed medication, because the drug itself "will get me addicted." This is never true. A drug may cause physiologic dependence and withdrawal symptoms when it is stopped—as demonstrated by the experience of a friend with cancer who developed "flu symptoms" after a hospitalization at a world-renowned cancer center. Upon discharge, her opioid pain medication had been discontinued abruptly; her runny nose, chills, malaise, and muscle aches were symptoms of opioid withdrawal, not a viral infection. Far more significant risk factors than the substance itself are a person's past experiences and family history that place the individual somewhere along the spectrum of risk for addiction.

We shall explore the development of addiction by looking at which factors create increased risk at each stage from initial use and experimentation through heavy use and addiction to remission and relapse. The clarity of this linear approach belies the complex interplay of forces in addiction and the distinctly nonlinear trajectory of individuals struggling with addiction and recovery.

The environmental influences of family and peers determine the age and circumstances of initial drug use. By adolescence, the behavior of older siblings and peers who use drugs carries more weight than parental admonishments or proscriptions (Linda). In contrast, the next phase of increasing experimentation derives from individual characteristics and behaviors, which reflect differences in brain systems involved in judgment and control of behavior. Youth with externalizing disorders (attention deficit hyperactivity disorder, oppositional defiant disorder, and conduct disorder) develop drug addiction at a younger age and have a more severe course of addiction than their more sanguine peers.[20] Traits of impulsivity and risk taking are linked to decreased activity in the pre-frontal cortex, an area involved in prioritization and decision making. This pattern of brain activity typical in adolescence is also seen in the brains of people with long histories of addiction. However, impulsivity is in no way specific for drug use, nor is a chaotic, unsupportive environment that fosters these traits.

Once a pattern of regular use is established, more addiction- and drug-related factors come into play. Positive reinforcement in terms of plea-surable experience drives escalation of use and the increasing salience of the drug. Among predictors of heavy use patterns as an adult, heavy use at age eighteen is more important than age of first use, adverse consequences from adolescent use, or deviant coping skills.[21]

Changes in neurotransmitters and receptors associated with addiction underlie its pattern of persistent, compulsive behaviors. These changes include the increasing prominence of memories related to drug use and the automatic behaviors triggered by those powerful memories. At the same time the brain's baseline level of dopamine (DA), the primary neuro-transmitter involved in addiction, is decreased, so that the DA system becomes hyperresponsive to drugs. In laboratory animals, these changes appear to increase the animals' motivation to self-administer an addictive drug.[22] Over time, these abnormal pathways become the default neural pathways, and all experiences are interpreted through the lens of addiction. Larry, for instance, was apt to think of heroin use and withdrawal.

Larry's first words were, "I feel like I'm withdrawing from dope [heroin]. I'm gonna need more Suboxone." Larry's opiate addiction had been in remission on a stable dose of Suboxone for four months; physical withdrawal was unlikely unless he had been using other drugs, which he denied. What was he feeling that made him think he was in withdrawal? His symptoms included feeling hot and cold with sweating, runny nose, sore throat, and cough; he felt anxious and restless, unable to focus or concentrate. What Larry was experiencing as withdrawal was more likely a common cold and the normal angst of being jilted by his current girlfriend—feelings he had avoided in the past by getting high.

Larry's emotional distress put him at high risk for relapse.[23] The neural pathways involved in a person's reaction to stress parallel neural pathways activated during drug use. His current stress was acute, but early adverse experiences and chronic stress had caused long-term changes in his brain's hippocampus and nucleus accumbens that also increased his vulnerability to relapse.[24] Not surprisingly, the longer a person has used drugs addictively, the more at risk he is for relapse, whether that susceptibility is a result of neurological factors (ingrained addiction pathways or underdeveloped brain regions involved in responsibility, decision making, and self-control) or truncated life experiences necessary to develop into a mature adult.

A less intuitive finding is that, in rats, a longer duration of remission from drug use appears to augment stress-induced relapse more than a shorter period of remission. These data seem to suggest that in some situations the disease of addiction will progress even without the use of drugs. While scientific research has not documented this pattern in people, long-term members of Alcoholics Anonymous have told me that when some people relapse after a remission of years, the severity of their illness is much worse than when they first stopped drinking. Such disease progression during a time of remission is certainly not universal. Unlike laboratory rats, many people with addiction develop the ability to mitigate their circumstances and protect themselves from future severe relapse. We are left with the question of whether these different outcomes reflect the differences between species in terms of neural pathways of addiction or rather a human being's potential to influence his environment and change the balance between vulnerability and resilience.

Bill returned several months after his first visit, telling me that his heroin addiction was worse than ever. The more he tried to stop his drug use, the more he needed to shoot up to deal with the fear and anxiety that he would never get sober. Starting him on Suboxone quelled the craving and drug use, but not his loathing and self-hatred. At age thirty-two, he was unemployed and living with his mother. Over the next four years he had many relapses, but they were getting shorter, and his visits with me more regular. Too self-conscious to walk into an AA meeting alone, Bill asked a cousin already in AA to take him to a meeting. Slowly, he engaged in AA, eventually attending meetings daily. He scraped together the funds to get a trucker's license and landed a job doing long-haul trucking. Always on the road, he did not have his AA support and had difficulty getting to my office for counseling and his Suboxone prescription. His Suboxone gave him headaches and nausea, so he decreased his dose, unmasking his cravings. Instead of relapsing, he quit his job and went back to his daily AA routine. He was hired by another company to make local deliveries. When Bill first started seeing me as a patient, his self-esteem was so low that I wondered if he could develop the strength to tackle his addiction. His determination, good judgment, and sense of agency surprised me.

Several neurobiological pathways appear to lead to relapse. In rats, emotional stress (in the form of foot shock) activates the brain's normal stress pathway with increased release of a hormone, corticotropin releasing factor. This hormone stimulates a complex neurohormonal system, the hypothalamic-pituitary adrenal axis (HPA), resulting in the increased output of hormones that mediate the common sensations of stress: anxiety, increased heart rate, and a sense of agitation and dis-ease—symptoms also common in drug withdrawal. Another route is the addictive pathway itself. A priming dose of a drug ("Just one drink won't hurt . . .") may trigger relapse in humans and laboratory animals.[25] More striking, because the phenomenon occurs in people determined not to use drugs, is the effect of drug-related cues. The unexpected sighting of a former drug dealer, the smell of marijuana smoke, the seductive whir of an ATM counting twenty-dollar bills may trigger an irresistible desire to use. Tapping into these drug-related memories leads virtually automatically to the behaviors needed to acquire, prepare, and use the substance.

A unique combination of forces from the genetic to the environmental level will determine whether a person with addiction relapses or resists the craving. Let us look first at the "internal" factors, those pertaining to the individual. To illustrate the complexity of these interactions, I shall describe genetic influences on molecular and cellular levels as they form biological systems. These processes underlie the personality traits, individual responses to stress, and psychiatric comorbidity that determine a person's vulnerability to addiction.

Genetic influences on a disease as complex as addiction are always mediated through a network of molecular and cellular systems that in concert lead to behaviors we recognize as addictive. To date, researchers have identified almost fifty different chromosomal regions associated with genetic vulnerability to addiction.[26] Some genes code for a specific biochemical product; many more influence the process of production—how much, how quickly, under what circumstances a gene product is produced. Multiple genes are involved, each having a modest effect.

Some genes have several different forms (polymorphism); these different forms, called alleles, confer relative vulnerability or protection in a given situation. An example is the effect of different alleles for serotonin, a major neurotransmitter, in response to childhood abuse. At low levels of abuse, children with genes coding for different serotonin alleles behaved similarly, but with a history of more severe childhood maltreatment, children with one allele were particularly vulnerable to depression, while those with another allele appeared protected. The children with a third allele had an intermediary response suggesting that this polymorphism of serotonin creates a spectrum of vulnerability.[27]

To complicate the picture, it is not only which allele a person has inherited but also the degree of penetrance—the degree to which that genotype is represented in its physical form (phenotype). Genes that code for a particular product are modulated by different sets of genes that determine quantitatively how much of this product is produced. This finding suggests an interesting question: Are disease states (high degree of penetrance) on a spectrum with no disease (very low penetrance) at the other end? In this scenario, it is the modulating genes that determine whether someone has a disease or not. Or, on the other hand, might there be a qualitatively different set of "disease-related" genes that exert pressure on modulating genes, implying that states of illness and health are discontinuous? Given the complexities of molecular genetics, the likely answer from research will be yes, both to these processes and to their interactions.

Drug use itself can induce vulnerabilities to drugs that are not seen in the non-drug-using population. The normal human brain has built-in systems that use neurotransmitters similar to opiates and to cannabinoids. Taking large amounts of these drugs appears to enhance the expression of polymorphism in genes that code for neurotransmitters and receptors in these systems.[28] As an example, adolescents with one form of an enzyme that breaks down neurotransmitters (catechol-O-methyl transferase—COMT) are at high risk of developing psychosis in the setting of heavy marijuana use, whereas adolescents with a different allele do not seem to be more susceptible even if they use marijuana heavily.[29] Perhaps not surprisingly, people with schizophrenia have a higher incidence of the COMT allele that increases risk for psychosis. The practical implication is that adolescents with family histories of psychotic illness need to know about their unique increased risks with heavy use of marijuana.

The different vulnerabilities related to alleles for COMT illustrate the highly specific origin of some vulnerability. On the other hand, inadequate coping skills in the face of drug use more likely reflect generic vulnerabilities rather than those related specifically to addiction. Low levels of the neurotransmitter serotonin are linked with impulsivity, aggression, and depression, all risk factors for antisocial behaviors as well as drug use. Novelty seeking and risk taking are associated with an allele coding for certain dopamine receptors. These receptors are widely distributed in the brain, particularly in areas associated with processing of attention, motivation, and emotion. This particular trait of novelty seeking appears linked specifically to the progression from drug abuse to dependence.[30] To complete the toxic cycle, acute intoxication and the chronic use of drugs impair the inhibitory control exerted by the prefrontal cortex (PFC) that might mitigate the heavy use of drugs.

Several major mental illnesses exhibit a similar decreased regulation by the frontal cortex. Post-traumatic stress disorder (PTSD) (Delia, Martha, and Linda) and attention deficit hyperactivity disorder (ADHD) (Larry and Delia) further decrease the inhibitory control of the PFC. Both PTSD and anxiety states increase the release of catecholamines, excitatory neurochemicals that create a hyperresponsive state. In schizophrenia, changes in the midbrain (hippocampus and nucleus accumbens) can lead to hyperresponsiveness to stimuli including drug use.[31]

People with addiction manifest extremely high levels of chronic personal stress. The emotional and physiologic experience of stress is expressed through the same brain pathways and mechanisms that are susceptible to addictive drugs. Repeated episodes of intoxication and withdrawal mimic repeated distressing events, leading to chronic stress reactions. The calming effect of sedative drugs like alcohol and opioids in the face of overwhelming anxiety and distress helps to perpetuate drug use. This was

Martha's downfall. When abstinent from alcohol, her anxiety, PTSD, and insomnia felt unbearable. Determined not to drink, she turned to prescription Xanax, a highly addictive benzodiazepine.

Whether biologically or pharmacologically based, precursors of this stress stem from genetic and environmental influences. The neurobiological pathways of stress and addiction have significant overlap. The feelings of acute emotional stress are familiar: anxiety, increased emotionality and sensitivity, feeling overwhelmed. Usual emotional defense mechanisms—distancing, rationalization, minimization—are of no avail. This hyperalertness and sense of danger are mediated through the dopamine systems and the hypothalamic pituitary adrenal axis (HPA), which translates mental stress into the associated hormonal and biological sensations mentioned earlier: increased alertness, muscle tension, rapid heartbeat, and raised blood pressure. In addition to the hormonal response, the brain responds to stress with an increased production of beta-endorphins (our own internal opiates), which may exert a calming effect.

Addictive drugs exert their effects on these same systems. Intoxication with cocaine or amphetamines activates the HPA system and releases increased amounts of norepinephrine, which impairs the brain's self-regulatory function (the anterior cingulate cortex and the PFC).[32] A decreased ability to monitor internal emotional and cognitive states and to modulate reward-related behaviors such as assessing future rewards, creating expectancy, and prioritizing activities can precipitate further drug use or other maladaptive behaviors. Observations in animal studies and in humans confirm that chronic stress in early life causes long-term changes in an individual's stress responsiveness that can impair resilience and increase vulnerability to drug use later in life.[33]

The happenstance of one's birth and the circumstances of childhood shape the genetic expression of personal development. Individual gene differences exhibit greater variation among those individuals with greater resources than those with fewer resources. The risks related to poverty of all kinds can overwhelm a genetic expression of strength.[34] As we have discussed earlier, a positive attachment between parent/caregiver and young child appears to be the major force in the development of resilience traits.

The critical nature of this relationship is demonstrated in a study of Romanian orphans adopted into middle-class British homes. These orphans, warehoused in large impersonal settings, were victims of the bizarre social policies of then-dictator Nicolae Ceauşescu. Those children who had spent eighteen or fewer months in the orphanage met normal developmental milestones by age eleven, whereas those children with twenty-four to forty-two months in the orphanage manifested significant developmental delay at age eleven.[35] The considerable social and economic resources of their adoptive families did not offset the earlier damage. Because each successive developmental stage is built on the prior stages, the foundation laid down in infancy assumes a critical importance.

Many environmental effects on a young child are expressed through relationships with parents or other primary caregivers. Parents can mediate social pressures in their roles as teachers, providers, socializers, and protectors.[36] Characteristics associated with a negative impact on children include maternal depression and anxiety, a low level of educational attainment, being a single parent, and a paucity of positive mother-infant interactions.[37] The negative effects of poverty are expressed through the mother-child relationship in myriad ways, such as the availability of food, levels of parental stress, and inconsistency of the family environment. Large family size with an unskilled head of household, being part of a disadvantaged minority group, and a rigid parenting style all militated against a child developing resilience. The loss of a parent through death or separation can deal a devastating blow to a child's resiliency. For Larry, his mother's death and his absent father increased his vulnerability. The pain of being without any family on Thanksgiving overwhelmed his resolve. He injected heroin once to numb his sadness and loneliness. On the positive side, Professor Rutter summarizes the qualities that promote the development of resilience: secure attachment relationships, harmonious relationships with extended family and close friends, opportunities to cope successfully with the challenges of adverse situations at different developmental levels.[38]

Parents with addiction affect their offspring by the environment they create in addition to the genetic material they pass on. A household with an addicted parent may expose a child to the stressors of family disruption, inconsistent parenting, internalized shame and guilt, or more blatant abuse and neglect.[39] Studies of twins and adopted children have demonstrated repeatedly that children of addicted parents have an inherited risk for addiction apart from any environmental exposure.[40] A well-known example is the increased risk for sociopathy and early onset addiction in sons whose fathers have those problems.[41] A person having a first-degree relative (parent, sibling, or child) with addiction has a significantly higher risk of developing addiction than someone without such a family history.

Linda is the thirty-three-year-old single mother who had used opiates and cocaine for many years. She came to me seeking office-based opiate treatment. She had grown up in poverty with two older sisters. Her mother was actively addicted to heroin and nicotine, and her father had bipolar disorder. Linda describes the household as chaotic with minimal parenting. Initially, she did well in school, but by age ten she was smoking cigarettes and marijuana.

In her first ten years, Linda had exposure to many more of the risk factors than the protective factors described in research literature. Before she was born, she was exposed to nicotine, possibly leading to lower birth weight. Infant-parent attachment is crucial for self-esteem and confidence;[42] the quality of her parenting was likely inconsistent given her mother's addiction and father's active mental illness, although the parenting provided by her older sisters may have mitigated that risk factor. Her memories of positive elementary school experiences may indicate a time of positive self-esteem and competence, which is a predictor of future competence. Her childhood world was confined to the bleakness of an inner-city housing project. She does not remember ever visiting the library, a museum, or the zoo.

During adolescence, peer influences eclipse family attitudes. Experimenting with new and risky behaviors is a developmentally appropriate task. The CRAFFT, a screening test for teens, succinctly captures worrisome behaviors associated with substance use (table 4.1).[43] It asks about risky behaviors (drinking or using drugs alone or to fit in), environmental risks (riding in a car driven by someone who has been using), and consequences of use (concern from family and friends, forgetting what happened, or getting into trouble while using). The CRAFFT questionnaire

Table 4.1 CRAFFT Questions

C	Have you ever ridden in a **CAR** driven by someone (including yourself) who was "high" or had been using alcohol or drugs?
R	Do you ever use alcohol or drugs to **RELAX**, feel better about yourself, or fit in?
A	Do you ever use alcohol or drugs while you are by yourself, or **ALONE**?
F	Do you ever **FORGET** things you did while using alcohol or drugs?
F	Do your **FAMILY** or **FRIENDS** ever tell you that you should cut down on your drinking or drug use?
T	Have you ever gotten into **TROUBLE** while you were using alcohol or drugs?

Source: © Boston Children's Hospital, 2013, all rights reserved. Reproduced with permission.

Note: Two or more "yes" answers indicate possible alcohol or drug problems and require further assessment.

was not designed to diagnose addiction in teens but rather to screen for risky behavior *related to* any alcohol or drug use along the spectrum from casual experimenting to addictive disease. In more recent work, the group that developed CRAFFT found that approximately 10 percent of teens with positive results on the CRAFFT score positive for substance use disorders.[44]

Adolescents who develop addiction may not have the emotional maturity or cognitive skills to achieve a lasting remission. Persistent intoxication through adolescence decreases educational attainment and thwarts the development of interpersonal skills required for positive intimate relationships or success in the work environment.

Those who have grown up in an addicted family do not have normal developmental building blocks on which to mature. Lack of positive early childhood nurturing leads to poor self-esteem, lack of confidence, and lack of agency. Addictive parents, with their own developmental challenges, may have modeled immature coping skills such as resolving conflict through violence rather than negotiation. The self-absorbed, impulsive behavior of an addicted person in his early twenties may reveal the emotional maturity of a thirteen-year-old boy.

Unable to tolerate living in a shelter, Larry had moved in with his new girl-friend and her two-year-old son. Unemployed, bored, and frustrated, he took a handful of pills offered by an acquaintance. He ended up in a hospital Emergency Department after having a seizure in front of the child. Child protective services were notified to investigate and monitor the home situation. Told by the social worker that he had to move out, Larry blamed his girlfriend and the hospital for his situation, "She didn't have to call 911, and the jerks in the ED overreacted."

Larry's response to his boredom is both maladaptive and understandable. He feels he has no control over his life and therefore abdicates all responsibility for his behavior. His lack of agency has some basis in reality; his history of addiction, a criminal record, and a tenth-grade education make him marginally employable.

Unfortunately, many people addicted in adolescence do not outgrow their addictive behavior. Not only are addicted people lacking in basic skills; they also have developed a highly maladaptive way of responding to their environment, for which drugs seem the perfect short-term response. Active addiction focuses solely on finding, preparing, and using a drug, and then recovering from its effects. This single-mindedness teaches and reinforces maladaptive skills. Desperation for the drug fosters ruthless behavior; lying, stealing, taking advantage of family and friends are all subsumed under the supreme value of a drug reward. Manipulation of others becomes a way of life that is hard to give up even in remission.

MK, a new patient referred by Larry, requested office-based opiate treatment with the understanding that she would be switching all her care to my hospital network and me. Her demeanor was sincere and serious about her recovery. Her urine drug screens were frequently positive for an anxiety medication that I was prescribing. After she showed up in an Emergency Department in another hospital system twice for overdoses of Suboxone and her anxiety medication, I learned from her former psychiatrist that MK had been getting prescriptions from both of us. She was apologetic and tearfully begged me not to stop prescribing Suboxone for her, saying that she would do anything to help her get her addiction into remission. We worked out some stringent limits: she would get her prescriptions only at weekly scheduled appointments; there would be no early refills of her medication for any reason, even if she came with a police report of loss or theft; she would engage in a more intensive outpatient treatment program.

A few months later, MK missed her appointment with me. She called sobbing, saying that she had been robbed at gunpoint and then sexually assaulted; all her medication had been stolen. I told her to come see me the next day.

When my patient arrived, her eyes were swollen and puffy; she was not wearing her usual makeup. She seemed withdrawn. In a hesitating voice, she described a brutal sexual assault. But no, she had not reported this to the police or gone to an emergency department; she had felt too ashamed and scared. And what was she doing in that deserted commercial neighborhood at that late hour? Her car had broken down on her way home from her boyfriend's apartment, and she was walking toward a gas station when this person came up behind her and stuck a gun in her back. How had she gotten home from the deserted commercial neighborhood where she had been attacked? The attacker hadn't gotten her cell phone, so she was able to call her mother to come and get her.

MK had an answer for everything. My skepticism and compassion were at war. Frankly, I didn't believe her story, and yet, if she had been assaulted, to deny her treatment for sexually transmitted diseases and rape counseling would have been inhumane. The acute trauma certainly put her at increased risk for relapse to opiates. I gave MK a prescription for a few Suboxone and asked her to return the following day. By the time all her treatment had been set up, her fifteen-minute appointment had lasted an hour. I was seething, feeling that I had been duped and manipulated and had inconvenienced all my waiting patients. By the time I learned two months later that the whole story was a fabrication, I felt more sadness than anger. MK's intelligence, her social skills, her own values had been subsumed by her addiction. For her to get well, she will need more intensive structured treatment than I can offer in my primary care office. I hope she makes it.

A marked change in drug use and behavior occurs among people in their mid- to late twenties. The proportion of heavy users and those whose behavior in their early twenties met criteria for substance abuse or dependence plummets from about 50 percent to the expected prevalence in the adult population of about 10 percent.[45] The decrease in drug use and the personal and social changes at this stage of development reflect the final maturity of human brain growth and frequently a change in social circumstance. Marriage, family, and employment are all sobering influences, often described as the "turning point" in recovery. Could these "turning points" be in fact the "tipping points"[46] that favor resilience over vulnerabilities? To consolidate their sobriety, some men in Vaillant's longitudinal study credited an alternative addiction: compulsive exercise, immersion in Alcoholics Anonymous (AA), or finding another more socially acceptable outlet for their addictive behavior.

Other users are not so resilient. Among this more vulnerable population, low self-esteem is a hallmark of addiction. Societal attitudes about addiction confirm the sense of failure.

Bill described repeated episodes of treatment, relapse, and more treatment as proof of his overwhelming failure, rather than evidence of his tenacious efforts to try to get off drugs. His pervasive negative self-perception prevented him from recognizing and building on the strengths that he had. He resorted to blaming others for his predicament: his homelessness was his girlfriend's fault; he missed his appointment because the receptionist told him the wrong date; he was asked to leave a treatment program after an angry outburst because the counselor was too sensitive. Bill had not accepted responsibility for his behavior and its consequences. As long as he assigned control of his life to forces outside himself, there was no impetus to change his own behavior. His learned helplessness reinforced the sense of hopelessness. His prognosis for establishing a solid remission seemed guarded.

Contrast Bill with Linda, mother of two young daughters, now separated from her unsupportive addicted husband. She had started to feel desperate again. Her psychiatric and addictions treatments were working well for her, but she was being evicted. Unable to work because of her current medical problems and child care issues, she had no way to pay the rent. But Linda had a plan. She would try to get into a family shelter; as a homeless family, she and her daughters would be eligible sooner for housing assistance.

"Nobody's going to take care of me," she announced. "I'm learning—" the words came more slowly. "I'm learning that I have to be responsible for myself, for myself and my kids. That's the only thing that matters."

Ten months later her resilience was still there despite crushing circumstances. An exacerbation of her bipolar disorder required a hospitalization. Her
children again went to live with her aunt and uncle, who did not allow Linda
into their house. Linda was staying in a "wet" homeless shelter, surrounded
by intoxicated people. Out on the street by 6:30 a.m., she spent her days in the
public library looking for jobs on the Internet or trying to get permanent housing for herself and her children, going to health care appointments, or going to
an AA meeting. It was a dismal existence. When her despair overwhelmed her,
she occasionally used drugs. But her commitment was to remission, to getting
healthy enough to care for her children again, to fighting to get her life back.

Other addicted people living in this "wet" shelter had given up. One man
had been living there—going out during the day to drink, returning at
night to sleep it off—for over twenty years. Repeated failures to achieve
lasting sobriety had taught him that the safest life emotionally was one
without aspiration or hope, devoid of responsibilities and expectations.
Human relationships were too complicated; his "best friend," alcohol,
was always there and made no demands while slowly killing him. The
singer Bob Dylan got it right: "When you've got nothing, you've got nothing to lose."[47] The bonds that could have connected him to a human
community were frayed beyond repair. He would die of his addiction.

This man's plight is a reminder that the downward spiral of addiction
is as near as the next drink or injection. As my addicted patients start to
get better, they talk about their fears of failing again.

"I've come too far; I don't ever want to go back there." Martha, a petite,
middle-aged woman with her hair drawn back in a ponytail, was describing her
early abstinence. Her voice conveyed bravado more than confidence as she
listed all her recent treatments for alcohol dependence and her plans for the
future. She would be living in a sober house, attending several AA meetings
weekly, and was enrolled in a program to teach her computer and office skills.

Over the next several months, her levels of stress and anxiety increased
dramatically. "Everything is going so well," she said. "Why do I feel like I'm
going to pick up again?" The thought of relapsing—failing again—frightened
her, but the idea of success was worse.

Failure was a known experience, even offering the familiar comfort of alcohol-induced oblivion if her stress became overwhelming. The pressure to succeed did precipitate a relapse, and she disappeared from my practice for several months. When she returned to resume treatment, she reflected on her need to progress more slowly, to take her successes in incremental doses. "Getting better" meant learning to live successfully with her addiction, not trying to escape it. This time the confidence in her voice sounded real.

Despite their difficult personal circumstances, both Linda and Martha have demonstrated impressive resilience. What personal attributes make resilience more likely? Dr. Stuart T. Hauser and Dr. Joseph P. Allen addressed that question in their longitudinal study of sixty-seven adolescents with psychiatric problems serious enough to require hospitalization in a locked psychiatric ward. First interviewed while hospitalized, these children were interviewed periodically over the next ten years. Nine of them (13 percent of the group) were highly functional as young adults. In their book *Out of the Woods: Tales of Resilient Teens*, Hauser, Allen, and coauthor Eve Golden share the narratives of these nine former patients and try to make sense of the common elements that made them so resilient. Three attributes stood out: first, a sense of personal agency that they could affect the course of their lives; second, a capacity for self-reflection; and third, an investment in caring relationships. "These three characteristics—agency, looking inward, caring about relationships—of the resilient teens are essential aspects of competence in human social interaction. . . . These stories suggest that mastery of human emotional and social interaction may be the culmination of all other aspects of resilience."[48] We understand, sadly, that this mastery is exactly what so many addicted people lack.

Linda and Martha, both thoughtful women, have proceeded on divergent paths. Completing her high school equivalency exam while still living in the shelter, Linda has just finished her second year at a local community college. After eighteen homeless months, she finally did receive subsidized housing and has been reunited with her daughters. Being a single parent of two teenagers has been challenging, but she is very much involved in their lives. With her increasing confidence as a mother and her success at college, she is beginning to believe in her own sense of agency. Not that her life is easy—she still struggles with her depression and poverty. But she hasn't used any drugs, except tobacco, in over four years. Linda sees a future.

Over the last three years, Martha has wrestled with her anxiety from post-traumatic stress disorder (PTSD), despite working with a therapist and attending AA meetings. She has had to sever all connection with her son, terrified of his drug-addicted violence and manipulation. Unable to work because of her PTSD, she was surviving by "couch surfing" among sober friends from AA. When she felt the small amount of Klonopin (antianxiety medicine) that I had prescribed was not enough, she got prescriptions from other doctors and bought the medication off the street. Fortunately, her sober housemate insisted that Martha get addiction treatment if she wanted to continue living in the apartment. Martha completed a four-week treatment program. I told her that it really was not safe for me to continue prescribing the addictive antianxiety medication; she relapsed again to alcohol and pills and quickly entered a long-term addiction rehab program.

Six months later, she was wary about the severity of her addictions but felt energized to prevent another relapse. Living again with her sober friend, Martha started attending daily AA meetings, started taking better care of herself, and even tried to stop smoking. However, she also reconnected with a former psychiatrist and persuaded him to give her a low dose of the very medication that had precipitated her recent relapses. The strength of her resilience and the power of her addiction continue to fight for control of her life.

This chapter has addressed abstract concepts about vulnerability and increased risk as well as protective factors and resilience in the face of addiction; it is ending with stories of individuals struggling with addiction. This movement from the general to the particular underscores the main theme in this chapter. While all genetic effects are expressed through a person's environment, the individual genetic traits and the specific environmental circumstances create a unique individual response that is difficult to predict. For example, sickle-cell *trait*, a condition inherited from one parent, can confer protection from malaria and thus actually enhance one's well-being in malaria-rich areas of Africa; but sickle-cell *disease*, a condition arising when the same gene is inherited from each parent, causes profound anemia and painful "crises" in any environment, resulting in strokes, kidney damage, and recurrent pain. Such is the nature of the relativist gene-environment interactions, which are, of course, far more complex in the case of addictive behaviors, resilience, and relapse. However, we can draw some definite conclusions.

The quality of early infant-caregiver relationships has a profound effect (for better or worse) on a person's later development, including harmful drug use and addiction. A severe genetic defect or a very deprived environment can overwhelm even robust resilience factors, but often it is difficult to predict whether the interaction of genetic and environmental variables will result in protection or vulnerability. Adverse events in early childhood may lead to more resilient responses later in life or, conversely can contribute to heightened stress responses in adults. Such stress responses and aspects of addiction share similar neurobiologies, underscoring the reinforcing negative overlap of these two conditions.

To achieve and maintain a healthy remission from addiction, a person must do much more than simply stop using drugs. Not that abstinence is easy. We have discussed the social and familial factors that predispose to continued use. Abstinence is an essential first step away from that path. Learning how to keep oneself safe from cues that trigger overwhelming drug craving and relapse requires a lifetime of work for many. Active addiction tells us that the person's life is unbearably painful, that she feels powerless to control or change her condition, and that the future she envisions bears no hope. It is hard to imagine a more vulnerable state.

Developing the flexibility of resilience, building personal agency, and the capacity for reflection are key skills in the recovery process. Full remission is not simply abstinence but, more importantly, the ability to live and function in the world while managing a chronic illness. Addiction treatment in the broadest sense aims to keep addicted people safe until they can manage their own physical and emotional safety. The next chapter addresses the process of recovery and the realities of treatment for addiction in our country.

FIVE

RECOVERY

OWNING THE TREATMENT AND THE OUTCOMES

The issue of self-management is especially important for those
with chronic disease, where only the patient can be responsible
for his or her day-to-day care over the length of the illness. For
most of these people, self-management is a lifetime task.
——Kate R. Lorig and Halsted R. Holman

At our first meeting, eighteen-year-old Larry slouched into my office, barely
looked up when I greeted him, and sat with his attention focused on his shoe-
laces. Just completing a five-day inpatient detoxification for opiate addiction,
he had been referred for office-based opioid treatment. He had been using
opiates for three years since his mother died. That first day my fleeting maternal desire to hug him told me how alone and scared he felt. Over the next
three years, he had two relapses to ongoing heroin use. Twice he got himself
into long-term residential treatment; he did a six-week stint in jail for violating
probation. At twenty-two, his addiction was in remission again. Once or twice
a year when his anger or sadness overwhelmed him, he would inject heroin.
Over the next several years after separating from his long-term girlfriend, he
has stayed with different friends but does not have a home. He is completing a
training program in auto mechanics. His sadness and loneliness are palpable,
but he is not using drugs. Treatment failure or treatment success?

Many high-quality research studies document that treatment of addictions is effective.[1] This sweeping positive statement begs many questions.

What are the goals of treatment? The outcomes? And how are they measured? Since addiction can last years, how long are research subjects followed? Are certain treatments better for some people than for others?

To answer these questions we need first to check our illness paradigm. In an acute illness, like pneumonia, the patient reports cough, fever, headache, and green phlegm; the clinician asks more questions, examines the patient, perhaps obtains a chest X-ray, makes a diagnosis of pneumonia, and prescribes treatment. In three to four weeks the illness is over, and the patient cured. If we examine Larry's story through this lens, his treatment is a failure. He received several months of intensive residential treatment, and far from being "cured," he relapses. His therapeutic relationships with his primary care physician and his former therapist do not prevent his occasional use of drugs.

This model of illness as acute episodes prevailed during most of the twentieth century. Until the discovery of antibiotics in the 1940s, many people died of acute infections or their complications. Most cancers could not be diagnosed at an early stage until the advent of advanced imaging techniques in the last thirty years. Without chemotherapy or radiation therapy to eradicate the disease or prolong survival, many cancers were likely experienced as acute, inexorable illnesses leading to death. By the 1980s, many cancers, diabetes, and lung disease had joined heart disease as chronic illnesses with times of relative health and acute exacerbations (heart attack, recurrence of cancer, or respiratory failure). By 2010, chronic illnesses accounted for the top five leading causes of death for residents of the United States.[2]

Treatment of chronic illness focuses on management of symptoms and exacerbations, not on cure. Prevention of relapse or complications demands an understanding of the patient's life circumstances, the role played by the illness, and a proactive approach to care. As a primary care physician with many patients suffering from chronic illness, I try to help my patients achieve three broad goals:

1. To recognize their illness and accept responsibility for it and its consequences
2. To develop knowledge and skills to manage their illness[3]
3. To optimize their function as contributing members of society

This approach applies to patients with addiction or with diabetes, arthritis, heart disease, or depression. Often patients must cope with two or three chronic illnesses simultaneously. Heart disease patients often have elevated cholesterol, hypertension, and nicotine addiction. A majority of people with addiction have a second or third psychiatric diagnosis.[4]

Recognizing and accepting a chronic illness represents the most difficult step for many people, especially at a young age. A software developer in his midthirties, still savoring the invulnerability of youth, takes pride in his independence and healthy lifestyle, which are predicated on physical ability and mental competence. If his physician recommends taking medication for his asymptomatic, uncontrolled hypertension, the likely response is, "I'll take care of it myself" with more exercise, weight loss, less salt. In his eyes, these lifestyle changes—which require motivation, determination, discipline, and the ability to plan and follow through—are preferable to the symbolic surrender of swallowing a daily pill. And I would agree wholeheartedly that changing to healthier behaviors is a better option than taking a medication, even though he may need medication to control his blood pressure in the future. I also know that at some point he will realize that taking care of his hypertension has infiltrated many aspects of his daily life. He can no longer take his good health for granted; he needs to pay attention. Some people can carry this burden lightly; for others, the burden of managing a chronic illness weighs heavily indeed. Severity of illness, poverty, and social attitudes about the illness may be enough to bring the overburdened to their knees.

Acknowledging one's addiction is a particularly heavy load. It is but a nuance of emotion from accepting that one has the illness of addiction to being overwhelmed with guilt and shame for all the damage that the addiction has caused. Bill, Delia, and Martha all know that this painful shame can paralyze the most determined efforts to care for oneself. Among my patients with other chronic illnesses, a more subtle shame drives the self-deprecation and confessions about not losing enough weight, not taking medications as prescribed. They find themselves caught in the contradiction between their professed value of "my health is the most important thing" and behaviors that suggest otherwise. Although certain behaviors may have contributed to their chronic medical illnesses, these patients do not identify with their disease to the same degree as do people with addiction and other mental illnesses. "Addiction is bad. I am an addict. Therefore, I am bad," is a recurrent theme among my addicted patients.

Learning to manage his hypertension while pursuing his career may not be challenging for our thirtysomething software developer. For an addicted person, these goals may seem unreachable. Why should this be? To start with, addiction is a "pediatric disease."[5] Drug use most often starts in adolescence, when children are testing their independence without benefit of the judgment and self-control of a mature adult brain. When an impulsive, emotionally volatile adolescent becomes addicted to drugs, his principal relationship is to that drug. His friendships and intimate relationships are subsumed by his addiction. The power of his addiction devalues family, school, and friendships and thwarts his ability to master the developmental tasks of adolescence. So there Larry sat, just discharged from a detoxification center, hoping for recovery—an eighteen-year-old man with the maturity of a fourteen-year-old. He could not learn to manage his addiction and function successfully in society until he had learned to manage himself.

Treatment for chronic illness requires treatment of the whole person, not simply his disease. The rest of this chapter will focus on treatment of the addicted *person*—the objectives of treatment and the process of recovery. We shall review treatment research looking at efficacy for achieving different outcomes. The chapter ends with a brief description of the addiction treatment system as a whole, its target population, its funding, and some ideas for the future of addictions treatment.

Treatment Objectives

Abstinence is the first objective of addictions treatment. The complete cessation of drug use is essential. An intoxicated person cannot participate meaningfully in treatment. Moreover, engaging someone in treatment for one addictive drug so that she can pursue her addiction to other drugs consumes important scarce resources. However, abstinence is never a sufficient outcome. While a primary treatment goal must be maintaining abstinence by teaching relapse prevention skills, successful programs simultaneously address limiting destructive behaviors and helping clients learn the cognitive and emotional skills they will need to manage their addictions and their lives.

For some severely addicted people with few internal and social resources, this goal of prolonged abstinence is not achievable. A decrease in the amount or frequency of drug use can be a reasonable goal. Harm reduction as an individual or public health goal for people with addiction has gained credence in the last decade, as there is increasing empirical evidence of its effectiveness.[6] As we understand more about the recurrent nature of addiction and the importance of limiting complications, attitudes about harm reduction have shifted. The cycle of craving a drug, searching for it, obtaining it, preparing it, using it, and recovering from it is an all-consuming pattern. Breaking that cycle, even partially, creates the possibility of a day or a week or longer in remission, an opportunity to learn how to protect oneself during the next relapse (e.g., learning not to drive while intoxicated or learning where to obtain free clean needles to prevent the spread of HIV infection), and perhaps a better chance for a shorter relapse the next time. The criticism of harm reduction is that on some level it condones drug use. The international evidence showing that harm reduction strategies in public health reduce HIV infection, increase participation in treatment, and decrease motor vehicle fatalities related to alcohol renders that criticism irrelevant.[7]

The process of extricating oneself from compulsive drug use forces the addicted person to address the destructive learned behaviors—lying, manipulating, committing violence against oneself and others—that help drive the compulsion. For the addicted person skilled in these maladaptive behaviors, there is a perverse pride in conning a doctor to write a prescription for pain meds. But then comes the guilt and shame of having stolen from families or friends who were trying to help. More painful still is the disgust and humiliation of those, mostly women, who have degraded themselves and their bodies to obtain their desperately needed drug. Even after working with me for years, these patients are too ashamed to speak aloud what they have experienced.

Lying and dishonesty are recurrent themes with my drug-addicted patients. A patient will tell me "Never trust an addict; we are all liars," but this time "I'm going to be honest with you, Dr. Barnes. You've really got to trust me." I have to remind them that I understand deception is a necessary skill for maintaining an addiction. Lying to me hurts only them. I measure my patients' progress by their behavior, not their words.

These first two treatment objectives, not using drugs and curtailing destructive behaviors, require a degree of emotional control and self-denial that many addicted people do not have. Some of my patients have taken the initiative to find, or family members may have insisted on, treatment that provides more supervision. I am impressed that many patients seem to find the degree of supervision that they need. Two of my young adult patients, both with significant histories of emotional trauma, opted for highly structured daily methadone maintenance treatment after more than two years of taking Suboxone. As one of them put it, "Now I have something to get up for every morning." Sometimes the recognition of a need for supervision is not enough, and the criminal justice system may force them into treatment. Two months after MC had told me that he hated using drugs and wanted to stop more than anything, the police found him with a needle in his arm in an open car parked in a public lot. He had never been arrested before. A suspended sentence and probation gave him much-needed temporary supervision. Since that time, he has not used opiates, and has found and kept a full-time job. With his wife and two-year-old child, he has moved away from his old neighborhood. Occasionally he uses marijuana, but he now inhabits mainstream society and not the drug culture. In retrospect, his blatant drug use seems to have been a cry for help.

The other treatment objectives—learning to prevent relapse, and developing the skills to manage chronic illness while building healthy emotional and interpersonal skills—are lifelong endeavors. Formal addiction treatment, measured in weeks or months, barely has time to help lay the foundation.

Relapse to drug-using behavior after years of abstinence puzzled addictionologists for many years. In the 1970s, the work of Dr. G. Alan Marlatt, a research psychologist in alcohol dependence, conceptualized relapse as a conditioned maladaptive response to high-risk situations that should respond to cognitive behavioral treatment.[8] Later research by him and his colleagues and more recent neuroimaging have confirmed this thesis. Relapse prevention, a mainstay of treatment, involves identifying the triggers or cues that may precipitate relapse. Certain internal or external cues can unleash a set of habitual behaviors that lead to using the drug. Addicted persons can usually identify these external triggers easily—my drinking buddies, seeing my drug dealer on the street, the smell of marijuana smoke, visiting the family—and try to avoid them. The internal emotional cues are more difficult to manage; chronic stress is part of an addicted person's daily life. When anxiety, trouble sleeping, and anger seem unbearable, the person with addiction knows that the only guaranteed way to relieve them is to take the drug, which is exactly what the person is trying to avoid. Many years ago, I interviewed a young woman going through a medical detoxification from opiates. In a monotone, she related that her father had died in a car crash when she was young, eighteen months ago her only sibling had died of a drug overdose, and six months later her mother died of alcoholic liver cirrhosis. Her recent relapse was triggered by the death of her boyfriend, killed in a drug deal gone bad. She was alone, unemployed, and homeless. Moved by her unimaginable losses, I felt my eyes stinging with tears, and I remember thinking to myself that she ought to just start using drugs again. Her life seemed too unbearable to live in.

Stress is a universal and necessary human experience. While driving on a crowded freeway, we protect ourselves by becoming more alert, attentive, and unable to relax. Chronic stress does not serve us so well. We may feel overwhelmed, angry, and unable to think clearly. Most of us have felt the telltale symptoms of stress: the knot in the stomach, the tension headache, or a clenched jaw. For the addicted person, stress is chronic and unrelenting, creating a permanent state of distrust and hypervigilance. The uncomfortable emotions of anger, sadness, anxiety, and depression may be particularly difficult to tolerate. Feelings of stress, common to most people struggling with addiction, share many brain pathways with addictive drugs and can trigger intense craving for a drug.

Acute craving for a drug lasts only a few minutes, although it feels as if the craving will intensify until satisfied by drug use. If drugs are immediately available, such craving is very difficult to resist. Once a person knows that this kind of craving is self-limited, the strategies of trying to distract oneself and of not having drugs available nearby can help a person get through an episode of craving. The ability to say no when offered a drug develops over time as the person learns to control impulsivity and to appreciate the potential consequences of relapse. The most effective approach to relapse prevention is to avoid any situation that might trigger craving. This task is particularly difficult to accomplish if a newly sober person has to return to her old neighborhood and drug-using acquaintances.

Delia learned this the hard way. After a year off drugs, she visited a supposedly sober friend who surprised her by offering some heroin, triggering intense craving. They ended up injecting the drug. In that episode, she contracted hepatitis C, a fate that she had avoided in over five years of prior injection drug use. She still cannot trust herself around any of her former drug-using friends.

Bill had an equally unexpected relapse. He was sitting home alone, annoyed that a friend had not called him as promised. Bored and restless, he decided to go out to get a soda. Just beyond the corner convenience store was a bar that he used to frequent, so he thought he would go there, but just to get a soda. Several hours later he stumbled home intoxicated from alcohol and cocaine. When did Bill relapse? When he picked up his first beer or sooner? He did not describe any positive craving for alcohol or cocaine. Most likely his relapse was triggered by the negative feelings of boredom and anger, followed by several poor decisions that seemed reasonable to him at the time. As he described this incident to me, Bill was incredulous that he had made those choices. The insidious power of craving had distorted his thinking, and he did not yet have the tools to see it coming. Members of Alcoholics Anonymous succinctly describe this distortion as "stinkin' thinkin'."

Perhaps the most important treatment objective is the development of healthy emotional and interpersonal skills. For people whose addiction started during their teen years, this process is essentially maturation from adolescence to adulthood. Because most people with addictions to alcohol, heroin, and cocaine have another psychiatric diagnosis[9] or a history of significant early psychological trauma,[10] there is additional healing needed. The developmental tasks of adolescence include responsibility for one's own actions and their consequences, regulation of impulse and emotion, development of peer relationships/separation from family, development of intimate relationships, capacity for self-reflection, and development of self-efficacy (agency). Certain cognitive functions also develop during adolescence: the ability to solve problems and make decisions, and the capacity for empathy and emotional flexibility. The last objective of addiction treatment is to develop cognitive and emotional skills to manage a chronic disease. Recent treatments for diabetes suggest that diabetic patients who learned how to manage their blood sugar levels and adjust their diets and insulin doses had improved diabetes control compared with a group less involved in their own treatment.[11] This investment in one's health can pay dividends in improved self-control and self-esteem.

How does this apply to Larry? His addiction is certainly chronic and the process of learning and relearning the skills to keep himself safe from relapse, painfully slow. His initial treatment goals were to stay off drugs and control the behaviors that kept getting him in trouble. Once the daily struggle to avoid drugs did not require all his energy, Larry discovered that he had a future. He dared to hope: He wanted to learn to manage his anger, regain his self-confidence, finish school, and get a job. He wanted a better relationship with his girlfriend, whom he wistfully called his fiancée. The noted Brazilian educator Paulo Freire recognized the importance of hope in his essay "Impossible to Exist without Dreams." He urged the educator, which is, after all, one of a physician's principal roles, "to create a context in which people can question the fatalistic perceptions of the circumstances they find themselves in."[12]

Like most of us, when Larry gets caught up in dreaming too much about his future, something right in front of him trips him up. When Larry had only a few months of recovery, another young man passed him on a crowded sidewalk and inadvertently jostled him. Furious at this presumed affront, Larry grabbed the young man by his jacket, raised his fist to punch him in the face, and stopped. His left hand released its grip on the other man's jacket, letting him fall awkwardly onto the pavement. Larry turned around and walked away quickly. "I could've killed him"—his voice betrayed wonderment and fear as he told me the story—"but I'm not that kind of person. And I didn't use." He paused. "I don't want to hurt anyone."

During his first few visits five years earlier, Larry had come across as a sweet, lost teenage boy who said he wanted to stay off drugs but didn't have any idea how to go about it. Essentially alone since age fifteen, when his mother had died suddenly, he had bounced around between his distant father's apartment and his grandmother's home. He soon found that opioid prescription drugs could ease the pain and loneliness of losing his mother, the major support in his life. A high school dropout, he spent his days doing a few chores for his grandmother and hanging out with friends or more often by himself. The Suboxone that I prescribed, he said, made him feel normal. And then he did not show up for his next appointment.

Several months later he returned from a residential rehabilitation stay, saying that now he realized that staying off the drugs wasn't easy and would take more work. He had found a therapist who helped him obtain disability benefits for his depression; he decided that he and his girlfriend, also in early remission from addiction, shouldn't live together, because it was too likely to lead to drug use. Sure that he would not fit in, but having no alternatives, he went to live at a sober house. Ready to defend himself against any slight, he complained that the staff seemed to punish him more than other residents involved in arguments and fights, but slowly the message of personal responsibility sank in. When asked to leave the residence after an argument that turned physical, he was able to acknowledge that the staff was just enforcing the rules and that it was up to him to keep his anger under control. He found and completed an anger management class. When he had a single lapse to opiate use, he learned to think about the incident as an opportunity to learn something new about how to keep himself safe and not as an excuse to keep on using. In the process of relapse prevention, he was doing a lot of the growing up he had missed during those crucial late teen-age years: learning how to control his emotions and to negotiate relationships with other people.

The Process of Recovery

Managing any chronic illness requires certain skills. Cognitive skills, the ability to understand the illness and its effective management, are essential. More important is the patient's sense of responsibility for taking care of the illness. The capacity for self-reflection—why is it hard? what are my goals?—enables a person to understand internal barriers and sources of strength. In behavioral terms, the person must be able to solve problems, make decisions, utilize available resources, plan, perform, and revise an action.[13] Fortunately, these are teachable skills. The acquisition of these life skills, which a successful or mature person might take for granted, builds the foundation of personal agency or "self-efficacy."[14] No longer is an addicted person's motivation just wishful thinking: "I really *want* to get off drugs"; it becomes the guiding purpose for a person who *can* get off drugs and start rebuilding his life.

MS, a sixty-two-year-old non-English-speaking woman with a third-grade education, managed her diabetes mostly by ignoring it. She did take her diabetes medications when she could afford them, but my brief attempts to educate her about this complex illness were met with smiles, vigorous nods of her head, and protestations that she knew what to do. Her blood test results said otherwise. After three visits with a nutritionist, MS returned with an entirely new outlook. She now understood the connection between her diet, her amount of activity, and her blood sugar levels. Instead of a vague response, she was eager to tell me what she had been eating and that she could predict whether her blood sugar would be better or worse. She was energized by this element of control over her health. More than the relationship between carbohydrates and high blood sugar levels, the nutritionist had taught her that she could control and manage her illness.

In *Pedagogy of the Oppressed,* Paulo Freire talks about this sense of agency or self-efficacy as a principal goal of education. The ability to understand and to change one's world becomes possible only if one can see oneself as separate from the world and with the ability to transform one's circumstances.[15] Bill, who had portrayed himself as a victim of circumstance and heroin for several years after starting Suboxone, now is working and surrounded by support from his AA community. Last week, he asked me about getting treatment for his chronic hepatitis C, a disease he had once described as "what I deserve for becoming an addict."

The current emphasis on improving the person's health, achieving remission, reducing harm, and preventing relapse or exacerbations of chronic illness has occasioned a major change in the patient-physician relationship. Most immediately notable is the shift from the powerful physician who prescribes and orders to the clinician who forms a partnership with the patient. No longer does the physician have both the authority and the responsibility for taking care of this disease; in the outpatient setting, the responsibility for managing the disease belongs to the patient, who in the best scenario develops the expertise and authority to care for herself.

Much of that care involves learning and reinforcing healthier behaviors. Changing behavior is a very difficult process and not one that the clinician can do for the patient. I have no illusion that I can exert any control over Bill's behavior after he leaves my office. The only person's behavior I can change is my own—so I have learned how to manage my behavior as a physician in order to help the patient explore her own motivation for achieving the behavior change she needs and learning ways to make it happen. I need to normalize the feeling that change is hard and uncomfortable, that change is predominantly a mental phenomenon, and that, once learned, the new behavior requires repetition and practice.

The concept of changing behavior is a recurrent theme in the treatment of addiction. Let's look more closely at the process of change, using the concrete example of an adult learning to ride a bicycle. Our nonrider has a lot of work to do before even getting on the bicycle. First, this person needs to have some dissatisfaction with the nonriding status quo: Taking the bus to work wastes too much time. My new boyfriend and all his friends are bike riders; I feel left out. I could really use the exercise. Then the doubts: Riding in the city is dangerous. I'll never keep up with my boyfriend anyway. A bicycle costs too much. Back and forth the person weighs the pros and cons of learning to ride a bicycle. Her friends try to help: the new boyfriend enthusiastically encourages her to learn, so she explains all the reasons why it is not a good idea. Her mother agrees: learning to ride a bicycle at her age is too dangerous. Perversely, her daughter explains that actually there are ways to ride safely; she'll buy a helmet, and anyhow, she wants to learn something new.

Now she is motivated; the positive reasons have outweighed the negatives. But how is she going to learn to ride a bicycle? Her eager boyfriend tells her that riding is so easy that she doesn't really have to learn and she should just go on a ride with him. Her mother suggests trying a very large tricycle first. Our soon-to-be rider settles on asking an old friend to teach her. This friend explains to her about balance and learning to fall and the use of the hand brakes. She is prepared to go.

She is riding! Ten yards, fifty yards! With her friend jogging alongside, she is terrified but exhilarated. She turns her head to tell her friend how much fun she is having; the bike skids on some gravel and she falls. More fearful than injured, she is reluctant to try again that day. Besides, she is exhausted from concentrating so hard on doing something new. Our friend has temporarily relapsed to nonriding behavior. After reconsidering the pros and cons, she decides to try again but now realizes that she'll need a lot of practice before she can call herself a bike rider.

Two psychologists, James Prochaska and Carlo DiClemente, in their work with smoking cessation, have described this process.[16] Based on observation, their "transtheoretical model of stages of change" captures the initial ambivalence as someone contemplates change, the importance of preparing for the change—wanting to change is not sufficient; one must also have planned how to effect the change—and then finally takes action. They describe six phases in the process of change: precontemplation, contemplation, preparation, action, maintenance, and relapse (fig. 5.1).

What these research psychologists understand is that ambivalence about current behavior is a necessary step, and relapse is a normal part of the change process. Most tobacco smokers require three to four attempts to quit before final success. The middle steps—contemplation, preparation, and action—require an uncomfortable degree of activation and commitment. A survey of outpatients with alcohol use disorders (AUD) in a medical clinic waiting area found that few people with AUD were actively engaged in change; most were in the lower-energy stages of precontemplation or maintenance.[17]

This change model can help us understand some of the more static concepts from Alcoholics Anonymous, such as being "in denial" or "having to hit rock bottom" before changing behavior. The psychological mechanism of denial, the refusal to acknowledge an unbearable truth despite overwhelming confirmatory evidence, is the hallmark of the stage of precontemplation. While initially an addicted person may be ignorant of the consequences of her behavior, more typically she knows

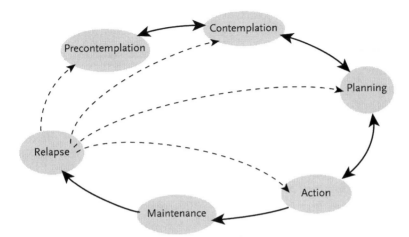

Fig. 5.1 Six observed stages in the process of changing behavior. Relapse is a normal part of learning a new behavior. From James O. Prochaska and Carlo C. DiClemente, "Stages and Process of Self Change in Smoking: Toward an Integrative Model of Change," *Journal of Consulting and Clinical Psychology* 51, 1983, American Psychological Association, adapted with permission.

on some level that there is a serious problem but is not able to admit to herself nor acknowledge to others the negative effects of her addictive behavior. After all, drug use seems like the solution to her misery, not the problem. Helping a patient to articulate the positive and then negative aspects of using or not using drugs may enable her to make a more rational decision about trying to change her behavior prior to catastrophic consequences or "hitting bottom." Denial plays a complicated role as someone tries to change behavior: denying that a problem exists, or that it needs fixing, can slow the change process down, but then denying (or not realizing) how difficult recovery is may give a person the courage to take the first step.

Learning to stop a behavior is more difficult than learning a new behavior. Ask anyone trying to give up smoking. Ask anyone who has tried to stop biting his fingernails or any young child who has had to give up a pacifier. Stopping those entrenched behaviors is always an act of courage. These dichotomous behaviors—you are using drugs or you are not— are easy to recognize.

Many other behaviors that addicted people need to address in recovery require prolonged attention. Consider Larry and his anger: even as he understood that he had to manage his own rage, he still needed the sober house and judicial system to set limits on his behavior. When Larry stopped himself from assaulting the pedestrian whom he thought had slighted him, he demonstrated a profound new sense of self-control. Would he behave the same way the next time? I hope that he would be able to tolerate his anger and not even turn around, but a more intense rage or less time to consider the consequences, and an impulsive assault, could land him back in jail.

As they pursue recovery, addicted people need to learn how to keep themselves safe emotionally. Having burst out of the cocoon of drugs, their raw emotions make them as fragile as a newly hatched butterfly. They are hungry to "get on with my life" but often not able to weather the change. Without self-confidence and competence to protect them, many people in recovery are one bad experience away from the deeply held conviction of worthlessness and failure.

Delia, the young woman who told me during our first visit that she had decisively severed all drug-related contacts by throwing out her old cell phone, has continued to struggle. She has worked in low-wage jobs trying to support herself and living alone in unfamiliar neighborhoods. She has survived a house fire and homelessness. She has tried repeatedly to get both psychiatric and addiction outpatient treatment. Her state-mandated health insurance does not cover the intensive program that seems right for her, and the covered programs have long waiting lists. She has come to my office discouraged and in tears but somehow managed to rally and leave with her Suboxone prescription and new determination. Then, unexpectedly, her manager fired her from her retail job. In her manager's voice, she heard her mother's comments echoing from childhood: she was no good, couldn't be trusted, looked too fat or too thin, couldn't hold a job. Delia was crushed by the familiarity of the self-loathing. Perhaps she really was "just an addict," and to prove her point, she relapsed. She pulled herself together, found a bed in a sober house, and committed again to her recovery. While she was struggling for economic survival, she was too busy and stressed to address the power of her addictions.

If the drug is no longer a trusted friend, to whom can an addicted person turn? This is a major problem for people with addiction, as many of their current "friends" are active drug users. Not until an actively drug-using friend comes by to chat and proceeds to steal all the medications in the bathroom cabinet do many people in early remission understand that addiction really is all about the drug and not about friendship. Other newly sober people are having their own struggles, which occasions a certain camaraderie, but these people, often on the cusp of relapse, are not necessarily more trustworthy. Former friends and family are wary; they have been burned before. Good treatment programs offer individual and group counseling that are usually time-limited because of inadequate resources. And what happens if the person in early remission relapses? The addiction treatment program may no longer be available, as abstinence is often a requirement for attendance.

Whether a person is using drugs or abstinent, Alcoholics Anonymous (AA) and other mutual-help groups, such as Narcotics Anonymous (NA) and AlAnon for families of people with addiction, provide a readily available community resource. AA is by far the most ubiquitous and accessible, with many meetings available every day of the week in metropolitan areas. The only criterion for membership in AA is a desire to stop drinking (and/or using drugs).

AA is a loose federation of individual groups whose sole purpose is to help its members stop drinking. Its principles are embodied in the Twelve Steps, guidelines for the spiritual and emotional growth of recovery, and Twelve Traditions, precepts aimed at keeping the AA fellowship free of outside influence, anonymous, and focused on its goal.

A preponderance of research from different disciplines has shown AA to be effective.[18] Six months' involvement in AA predicts abstinence up to sixteen years later.[19] In this study of some six hundred individuals seeking treatment, twice as many subjects attending AA (sixty-seven percent) were abstinent as compared to those not exposed to AA (thirty-four percent). Longer participation in AA increased the likelihood of abstinence in the future.

One caveat is that formal clinical trials comparing the effectiveness of AA versus other forms of treatment have had mixed results, suggesting that there may be common processes in AA and other treatments that account for the effectiveness of all over time. The cognitive precepts in AA most predictive of positive outcomes (commitment to abstinence, loyalty to the program, and avoidance of relapse triggers) inform other treatment

models as well.[20] In AA, the contemporary therapeutic processes of enhancing motivation, strengthening self-efficacy, bolstering active coping
skills, and providing opportunities to develop more adaptive social network skills were more indicative of improved outcomes than AA-specific
processes such as spirituality.[21] Affiliation with a mutual-help group following formal addiction treatment is associated with greater motivation
for sobriety, stronger sense of self-efficacy, and better coping skills—all
traits indicative of better outcomes.[22] Perhaps, those who choose to attend
these mutual-help programs are already the ones who have better internal
resources and social skills, who are more likely to do well no matter what
treatment.

My patients have had varied reactions to my suggestion that they attend AA or NA meetings. Martha and Bill have embraced the fellowship,
found sponsors within the program to help them with their recovery,
and have eventually become sponsors themselves. They typically attend
five to six meetings a week, plus take time to speak with their sponsors.
My patients who avoid these meetings describe anxiety being with other
people or sometimes the triggering effect of hearing another person talk
about drug use. They are often the patients who would most benefit from
the networks of people with stable sobriety that comprise an AA or NA
group. Larry, adrift since fifteen, attends an occasional meeting with
friends but is still too scared to take the risk of trusting other people. MC,
who never lost the support of her family, has thrived in AA, developing a
close relationship with her sponsor, attending intensive AA study groups,
and enjoying alcohol- and drug-free social activities with her AA friends.

Sometimes, by default, I become one of the most consistent figures in
these patients' lives, seeing them every month or two for over a decade. I
will see someone in abstinence or relapse, homeless or housed, employed
or not. Much of my work is simply to take the time to listen and to provide emotional support—celebrating every incremental step forward,
trying to reframe the self-contempt that there hasn't been more change
as instead an understanding of how hard these changes are, of how much
practice they take, and that, as more than one of my patients has told me,
"Any day without drugs is a good day."

Mostly I listen to the pain of the past and the frustrations of the present. In that listening space, some of these addicted patients express a new

capacity for self-reflection. I understand what William Carlos Williams meant when he spoke of the patient and physician creating together a completely new and unique moment: "The physician enjoys a wonderful opportunity actually to witness the words being born. Their actual colors and shapes are laid before him carrying their tiny burdens, which he is privileged to take into his care with their unspoiled newness. . . . No one else is present but the speaker and ourselves; we have been the words' very parents. Nothing is more moving."[23]

Perhaps most satisfying for me is watching these patients take the trust that they have learned from interacting with me and start to reach out to form new healthy relationships with people not using drugs. And while they will tell me that trusting someone else is the most difficult thing for them, I know that learning to trust themselves is even harder.

The Current System for Addiction Treatment

Amid all this struggle, where is the science to guide treatment decisions? First, we do know that treatment is better than no treatment, although few studies extend beyond twelve months.[24] However, a positive response to treatment at six months predicts a positive outcome in five years.[25] In a meta-analysis including over eight thousand people who sought addiction treatment, one-quarter of those attending more than one treatment session were abstinent from alcohol at one year and another 10 percent were using alcohol in a moderate and nonproblematic way. Second, for those who had relapsed to drinking, overall consumption decreased by 87 percent with a 60 percent decline in alcohol-related problems.[26] This large group of people who were still drinking but showed significant improvement is important. Such in-between results are often overlooked in the dichotomous paradigm of abstinence versus relapse. However, when viewed along the continuum of alcohol use disorders, such a decline in use and in associated problems indicates an overall positive prognosis.

Specialty addiction treatment settings provide intensive services to their clients. Larry and Delia have attended outpatient programs that offered individual and group counseling, often in the setting of an intensive two- to four-week daily program. Ideally these programs address clients' other mental health needs, which can significantly impede a client's ability to benefit from outpatient addiction services. Some larger programs also provide "wraparound" services of help with housing, vocational training, and disability determination. A large review of treatment programs over thirty years found clear evidence that treatment reduced substance use and crime.[27] A surprising finding was that no specific treatment method was superior to any other in its outcomes. Why should that be?

The common denominator of most treatment programs is engagement with therapists and with other people working to maintain their addictions in remission. Treatment can provide a safe "laboratory" to express difficult feelings and vulnerabilities. The quality of the relationship with the therapist may be more important than the particular counseling techniques. In a small but intriguing study, addicted clients whose counselor had an empathic style were significantly more likely to stay in treatment than those whose counselor was confrontational.[28]

Residential programs provide more structure and supervision. They also serve those who, because of homelessness or lack of income, have nowhere else to go. These programs range from two- to four-week intensive licensed inpatient treatment to halfway houses and unregulated sober houses where residents may stay for several months attending a prescribed number of AA or NA meetings weekly. The quality of the program and the readiness of the client vary considerably: Bill talked gratefully about the sense of security and safety of his most recent halfway house; CF, a young polysubstance abuser, railed about the excessive rules and the staff's attitude at a well-respected halfway house. Delia's relief at finally being in a secure sober house gave way to horror and trauma from bedbug infestations, roommates who stole from her, and other clients who were actively using drugs in this supposedly "sober" house.

The attitude of CF speaks to the common perception that coerced treatment is not effective. He had been mandated to the program by the court. However, some people, such as Larry, do seem to benefit from non-voluntary programs, although the evidence is not robust.[29] Coercion gets people into treatment and keeps them there, and treatment outcomes in terms of relapse and recidivism are similar for coerced and voluntary treatment.[30] Similar to the situation among clients with empathic, non-judgmental counselors, probation officers who were respectful of their clients, rather than confrontational and demeaning, had better outcomes with them.[31] Unfortunately, despite the high prevalence of people with addiction problems in the criminal justice, social welfare, and mental health systems, there is a significant absence of screening for addiction, let alone effective, compassionate treatment, due to an inadequately trained workforce.[32]

The national treatment system for addiction is inadequate and often substandard in the care delivered. A look at who pays for substance abuse and mental health care is instructive. Private health insurers, which are not required in many states to provide any mental health and addictions care, spend only 4 percent of their budgets on mental health and addictions, whereas addiction and mental health treatment uses up 30 percent of public resources spent on health care.[33] Despite the evidence that addictions care is cost-effective, some private health insurers do not include mental health and substance abuse care as covered benefits. The fact that the U.S. system ties health insurance to employment compounds the problem. When Delia lost her job, she lost her self-esteem and her benefits. When she relapsed and was too ill to work, she had to rely on public health insurance, which allowed her to continue to see me but not to attend the addictions program we thought would be most helpful. Linda has had a similar problem at her community mental health center. When her psychiatrist and longtime counselor left, Linda was promised another counselor and psychiatrist. Some two years later, she has not been assigned a psychiatrist, and the new counselor's inexperience and judgmental manner drove Linda away.

The underfunding of addictions care has led to a shortage of treatment programs, and those that exist often provide substandard care. Fewer than 15 percent of people with addiction ever receive specialty addictions care. Fewer than 11 percent of addiction programs provide care consistent with available scientific knowledge.[34] Most directors of addictions programs have bachelor's degrees or less than bachelor's-level education. Between a private system that has washed its hands of these patients and a public system that is underfunded, it is not surprising that needed addictions treatment is substandard or simply not available.

Larry's care has suffered from the consequences of underfunded addiction treatment; his care is fragmented, not coordinated, episodic (instead of long-term), and at times simply not available. He sees me for primary medical care and his Suboxone prescription. Rarely he attends NA meetings, but he has had to move so often that he has not found a comfortable and safe "home" NA group. For several months, he found housing through an agency that provided him with an apartment and some supervision in managing a budget and paying his bills. A brief relapse to drug use landed him back on the street, no longer eligible for the transitional help he so desperately needs. He has been unable to find mental health care for over two years. The psychiatric clinic in the public health system where I work cannot accommodate him, because of budget cuts. He has contacted several agencies in his current community and has an intake appointment in two weeks. Until he is housed, he cannot think about vocational training or finishing his high school education.

In the many cases when specialty addictions care simply is not available, where can people turn for treatment? My assertion that the primary care community setting is the best place to treat many people with these disorders may come as a surprise. Yet, in many important ways, addiction is a prototypical primary care illness. It involves the biological and psychosocial aspects of care. Addiction needs to be understood in the context of the patient's life circumstances. It is likely to require a combination of medical and psychosocial interventions.

Primary care clinicians provide an accessibility to care uncommon in other specialties. Almost any complaint can get a patient an appointment, and for me, this includes my addicted patients. I will see them whether their addiction is in remission or relapse (as long as they are not acutely intoxicated). I follow them for their other health problems and can maintain contact even when the person is not ready to change.

FL, a beefy man in his early forties, stated he had come to see me because his girlfriend wanted him to get a checkup. By the end of our first meeting, I had diagnosed hypertension, obesity, and alcohol addiction. "Nobody is going to tell me to stop drinking," was his retort to my concern about the several cases of beer that he drank weekly. When I assured him that my role was to give him the information about his health and not to tell him what to do, he reluctantly agreed to come back in a month for a blood pressure check. His blood pressure was still high; his alcohol use had not changed. At an appointment several months later, he had lost several pounds and his blood pressure was in good control. Almost casually, he reported that he had stopped drinking a month prior. He has not had a drink in almost three years.

PG, a laboratory technician in her late twenties, came in once a year for her annual checkup. She was healthy and had always denied any issues with alcohol or other drugs. I was standing behind her, one hand on her shoulder, listening to her lungs, when she whispered that she needed help to get off heroin. We worked to find her an evening program that would not interfere with her job. Like many young, high-functioning people with addiction, she had not accepted how serious her problem was. I have not seen her in over fifteen years; I hope that by now she has learned.

In the primary care office, we have the opportunity and obligation to screen for potentially harmful problems, including substance use. Just as a Pap smear screening may diagnose a precancerous condition and prevent cervical cancer, screening for substance use can prevent more serious problems by identifying people whose use puts them at risk for addiction. Screening also identifies people whose heavy use has already caused problems apart from the risk of addiction. In fact, the relatively large group of heavy drinkers accounts for a higher burden of social costs than the smaller group of addicted people.[35] The Institute of Medicine's recommendation to broaden the base of alcohol treatment to include a primary care foundation (fig. 5.2) acknowledged more than twenty years ago that the occasional accidents or days lost from work among many, many heavy drinkers far outweighed the many problems of the smaller number of people with addiction.

Effective interventions for substance use problems and for addiction are available to the primary care provider. Brief counseling sessions (five to fifteen minutes) by primary care physicians have decreased alcohol use significantly.[36] Further, this counseling has led to fewer hospitalizations, Emergency Department visits, and incarceration, accounting for a six-to-one cost savings to the community.[37] Not all brief interventions studied have had such impressive results, but brief interventions have been evaluated in many different countries and settings.[38] While many primary care physicians still feel uncomfortable screening for and

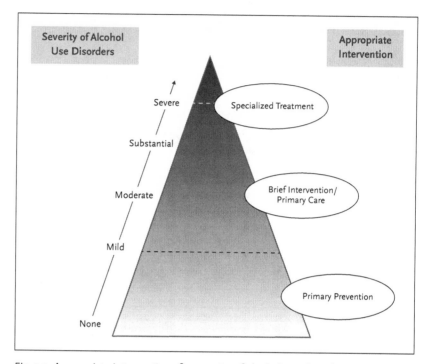

Fig. 5.2 Appropriate interventions for severity of alcohol use disorders. Reprinted with permission from *Broadening the Base of Treatment for Alcohol Problems*, 1990, by the National Academy of Sciences, courtesy of the National Academies Press, Washington, D.C.

addressing substance use problems, counseling about smoking and other health problems is slowly becoming an expected competency in primary care. Generalizing this expertise to other addictions is a logical next step.

As primary care practices redesign themselves as "patient-centered medical homes," they are becoming more proactive in caring for communities of patients with chronic illnesses in addition to caring for patients individually. Registries of patients with diabetes or depression have allowed more systematic outreach to those whose illnesses are not well controlled. Group visits of patients with similar problems and peer education have increased patients' self-efficacy and decreased costs.[39] Peer-led education groups for opiate-addicted clients resulted in a significant decrease in heroin use and injection risk behaviors.[40] These practice techniques are not yet considered standard-of-care for common

Table 5.1 The Quality Chasm's Ten Rules to Guide the Redesign of Health Care

Care based on continuous healing relationships	Patients should receive care whenever they need it and in many forms, not just face-to-face visits. This rule implies that the health care system should be responsive at all times (24 hours a day, every day) and that access to care should be provided over the Internet, by telephone, and by other means in addition to face-to-face visits.
Customization based on patient needs and values	The system of care should be designed to meet the most common types of needs but have the capability to respond to individual patient choices and preferences.
The patient as the source of control	Patients should be given the necessary information and the opportunity to exercise the degree of control they choose over health care decisions that affect them. The health system should be able to accommodate differences in patient preferences and encourage shared decision making.
Shared knowledge and the free flow of information	Patients should have unfettered access to their own medical information and to clinical knowledge. Clinicians and patients should communicate effectively and share information.
Evidence-based decision making	Patients should receive care based on the best available scientific knowledge. Care should not vary illogically from clinician to clinician or from place to place.
Safety as a system property	Patients should be safe from injury caused by the care system. Reducing risk and ensuring safety require greater attention to systems that help prevent and mitigate errors.

primary care problems, let alone substance use and addiction, but there are opportunities for primary care to be more active in identifying and managing patients with, and at risk for, addiction.

The Institute of Medicine has called for the redesign of health care and, in a 2006 report, for improving the quality of health care for mental

Table 5.1 (*Continued*)

The need for transparency	The health care system should make information available to patients and their families that allows them to make informed decisions when selecting a health plan, hospital, or clinical practice, or choosing among alternative treatments. This should include information describing the system's performance on safety, evidence-based practice, and patient satisfaction.
Anticipation of needs	The health system should anticipate patient needs, rather than simply reacting to events.
Continuous decrease in waste	The health system should not waste resources or patient time.
Cooperation among clinicians	Clinicians and institutions should actively collaborate and communicate to ensure an appropriate exchange of information and coordination of care.

Source: Reprinted with permission from *Crossing the Quality Chasm: A New Health System for the 21st Century*, 2001, by the National Academy of Sciences, courtesy of the National Academies Press, Washington, D.C.

health and substance abuse conditions.[41] Its ten-point program (table 5.1) would put Larry, Linda, Delia, Martha, and Bill at the center of a web of care with communication and cooperation among their providers and adequate resources for them to get the appropriate care that they want and need. They would have access to mental health and addictions care at whatever levels their illness requires throughout its chronic course. The United States' health care system is far from meeting these ten rules; the addiction treatment system has even further to go.

I am optimistic that further research will continue to confirm the effectiveness of addictions treatment for patients and its cost-effectiveness for the country as a whole. New cost-effective methods such as brief interventions, early screening, and peer education are already available. There are two serious stumbling blocks: educating the health professions workforce and mustering the political will to fund care for these patients.

There have been significant efforts to train health professionals in screening and brief intervention for alcohol problems, as well as to increase the number of trained faculty.[42] Unfortunately, most health professions schools, still blinded by the social stigma of addiction, have not instituted this training.

Building political resolve will require education to dispel the misunderstandings and myths about addiction. It will also require the philosophical commitment to help those less fortunate than ourselves. As Franklin Delano Roosevelt challenged the nation in his Second Inaugural Address: "The test of our progress is not whether we add more to the abundance of those who have much; it is whether we provide enough for those who have too little."[43]

SIX

DRUGS FOR DRUGS

Martha had done well for almost a year after her positive experience in a halfway house, but today she looked sick. Her skin was clammy; her hand shook as she greeted me; her face was bloated and red. Tearfully, she reported that she had been drinking for about a month but had stopped completely two days ago. She felt anxious and nauseous, unable to sleep or eat, but she didn't want to treat herself buying Klonopin off the street and becoming readdicted to benzodiazepines (primary medications to treat alcohol withdrawal). She had already arranged to return to her halfway house but first needed treatment for her alcohol withdrawal. She had never had any serious complications related to alcohol withdrawal and had a good support system, so I prescribed her medications for an outpatient detoxification. That was three years ago. Today she is sober and active in AA, but there have been costs of inadequate income, housing insecurity, alcohol-related health problems, and the emotional loss of having to sever all connections with her addicted son.

Disgusted with himself and "dope sick," Bill could only see his failures. After missing an appointment with me, he had run out of his prescribed Suboxone and resorted to heroin use to stave off the worst symptoms of opiate withdrawal. Too ashamed to call my office to ask for a few days of his medication until he could see me, he had used heroin once, despite attending AA meetings and talking with his sponsor daily. What I saw was a man with such severe addiction that even the fear of withdrawal eclipsed his rational judgment and catapulted him into drug use. A man who did not want and no longer enjoyed using drugs. A man who had developed just enough of something—hope, self-belief, connection to his sponsor, his AA group, his doctor—not to go "back on the street" for weeks or months, as he had done so often in the past. This was evidence of tremendous growth for him, progress he confirmed by being able to tolerate my reframing this experience as more victory than failure.

Addiction to drugs involves repeated episodes of intoxication and withdrawal from the effects of the drug. When a person's addiction is in remission, there is always the threat of relapse to drug use. Medications are available to treat the potentially life-threatening effects of a drug overdose or severe withdrawal from drugs. These medications, used to keep people safe from the dangerous effects of drugs, contrast with those medications used to prevent relapse to drug use. As the science of addiction becomes more sophisticated, understanding of the specific neural pathways involved in addiction creates opportunities to develop medications aimed at specific targets in the brain that produce craving.

None of the medications available is a cure for addiction. These medications keep a person safe (abstinent and involved in medical treatment) and provide an important platform for addressing the emotional and behavioral issues that can precipitate relapse to drug use. Because of the psychological damage of addiction, psychosocial treatment (formal or informal) is the mainstay of treatment for many people. This chapter will first address the use of medications to keep people safe from the acute effects of intoxication and withdrawal from drugs, and then focus on the more promising area of relapse prevention.

Medications for Managing Acute Intoxication and Treating Withdrawal

Addictive drugs generally fall into two classes, depressants and stimulants, depending on their toxic effects. Depressants are sedating and at high doses may cause respiratory depression and death. Drugs in this category include alcohol, opioids, benzodiazepines, and other sedatives alone or, more dangerously, in combination. An acute overdose can easily occur, especially when the person is naive to the drug and the brain has not developed tolerance to cope with the sedative effects. The acute alcohol poisoning seen in a college student exposed to alcohol for the first time falls into this category. Opioid overdoses are more common, primarily because of the misuse of prescribed pain medications. Opioid-addicted people may not know the potency of the illicit drug they are using, or they may combine it with other sedative medications. A particularly vulnerable population are those recently released from prison, or someone like Jackie terminated from her methadone treatment, as they may have lost all their tolerance to opioids. If they take the same "dose" of opioid that they had been used to, it will likely cause a severe overdose and death. In this country, there is currently an epidemic of overdoses from heroin and prescription opioids such as oxycodone. As of 2010, the approximately 36,000 people dying yearly from drug overdoses (primarily from prescription drugs) has exceeded the number of all motor vehicle fatalities annually.[1] And remember that a significant number of those motor vehicle crashes involve people intoxicated with alcohol or other drugs.

For opioid overdoses, there is a direct antagonist medication that displaces the opioid from opiate receptors. This medication, naloxone, has widespread use in emergency departments for patients brought in comatose. A positive response to naloxone (waking up) confirms that the patient's problem includes at least an opioid overdose. Since most overdoses occur in the community, often among other people using drugs, there has been increased interest in making this medication available to opioid-addicted people. Currently, a nasal spray form of naloxone is available and has been promoted in some communities around the country. Between 1996 and 2010, over fifty thousand people were trained to administer naloxone with a reported reversal of ten thousand opioid overdoses.[2] This form of harm reduction needs to be more widely available.

Unfortunately, there are no specific antidotes to overdoses with alcohol or other sedatives. Emergency care includes protecting the person's airway from aspiration of saliva and vomit and, if the overdose is severe enough, mechanical ventilation on a respirator until the effects of the drug wear off. Just letting an intoxicated friend "sleep it off" can be a life-threatening decision.

The effects of severe stimulant intoxication pose different problems. The most well-known drugs in this class are cocaine and the amphetamines. Initially, intoxication is activating, hence the nickname "speed"; there is an increased sense of well-being, or personal power, often accompanied by heightened physical activity (staying up for days at a time) and sexual energy. These drugs release the potent neurotransmitter norepinephrine, which causes constriction of blood vessels and can lead acutely to heart attacks and strokes. Within days of his 1986 first-round draft pick by the Boston Celtics, star college basketball player Len Bias succumbed to a cardiac arrhythmia at age twenty-two due to acute cocaine use.[3] As people become addicted to stimulants, they may binge on these drugs, using them around the clock until the supply runs out or they are too physically exhausted to continue. As these people start to withdraw, they can become highly agitated and paranoid that those around them are actually trying to harm them. They are a danger to themselves and others. The medical treatment involves using sedatives to calm them down until they fall asleep from exhaustion.

While acute overdoses occur in people both with and without addiction, withdrawal from the chronic effects of a drug is the hallmark of physical drug dependence.[4] As a person's brain becomes used to functioning while in a state of intoxication, the person develops tolerance to many of the drug's effects. This adaptation is mediated primarily by changes in brain circuits and neurotransmitters that blunt the effects of the drug. For instance, a person tolerant to the effects of alcohol may have a blood alcohol level several times the legal limit and yet superficially appear normal. In such cases, however, important neural pathways have been reregulated to offset the sedative effects of chronic alcohol ingestion. When the sedative drug is stopped for any reason, the increased outpouring of neurotransmitters causes overactivity of brain circuits and clinical manifestations known as withdrawal. The severity of alcohol withdrawal ranges from mild to life threatening. Early symptoms include anxiety, sweating, shakiness, nausea, vomiting, and difficulty sleeping. In the more extreme forms of alcohol withdrawal, a person may develop seizures, severe agitation, hallucinations, disorientation, as well as rapid heart rate, high blood pressure, and fever. Because severe confusion and body tremors are among the most obvious symptoms, this syndrome is called delirium tremens or DTs. Development of the alcohol withdrawal syndrome is unpredictable from person to person. Of two people both drinking heavily for several weeks, one person may stop drinking with only mild discomfort while the other may require hospitalization. However, the severity of withdrawal predicts how much difficulty someone will have the next time he stops drinking.

Withdrawal from opioids produces a different syndrome. Common symptoms include malaise, flu-like symptoms, chills with arm and leg hairs becoming erect (hence the term "going cold turkey"), nausea, vomiting, abdominal cramps, diarrhea, and jerking movements of leg muscles ("kicking the habit"). Add to these symptoms severe anxiety and difficulty sleeping, and the opioid-addicted person is in for a very unpleasant few days. It is not surprising that the onset of withdrawal is a strong trigger to use drugs again to quell these symptoms.

Unlike sedative drugs, the stimulants do not produce dangerous withdrawal syndromes. After repeated use of a stimulant, the brain becomes depleted of dopamine. As the major transmitter in the brain's reward pathway, dopamine tells us whether an experience is better or worse than expected. A general decrease in dopamine availability means that everything seems worse than expected. People who stop using stimulants after daily or repeated binge use describe a lack of interest in life, no pleasure with any activities, fatigue, and decreased energy. These experiences make the future seem bleak indeed and fuel a desire to recapture the feelings of well-being that the drugs initially impart. Unfortunately, there are no medications to treat stimulant withdrawal. Even medications that promote dopamine availability in the brain, for instance medications used to treat Parkinson's disease or some types of antidepressants, have not been effective.

The treatment of alcohol, sedative, and opioid withdrawal syndromes follows two basic principles. The first is to reintoxicate the withdrawing patient with a medication that is cross-reactive (i.e., interacts with the same brain receptors) and then to taper that drug slowly to minimize the withdrawal symptoms and give the brain time to start adjusting to its new drug-free state. The second is to use a medication that is longer acting than the addicting drug. The body metabolizes alcohol rapidly, about one drink per hour, precipitating the withdrawal syndrome over just a few hours. By treating the patient with a medication with a much longer duration in the body, the symptoms occur more gradually and can be more easily managed. For alcohol, the commonly used medications are benzodiazepines, a class that includes medications for anxiety like Ativan or Valium. The most commonly abused opioids, prescription medications such as oxycodone, and heroin have half-lives of just a few hours. Methadone and buprenorphine, both with half-lives of at least twenty-four hours, are now used to treat opioid withdrawal. Methadone can be prescribed only in a hospital setting or a licensed methadone clinic, whereas buprenorphine has the advantage of being available in outpatient settings. Before buprenorphine was available for detoxification, opioid withdrawal was often treated with a set of medications that treated the symptoms of withdrawal but did not affect the underlying processes in the brain.

The astute reader may wonder why an addicted person does not just become addicted to the medications used for detoxification. While people with addiction can become addicted to several different classes of drugs, most of the detoxification medications are not very desirable. As Dr. Mary Jeanne Kreek, head of Rockefeller University's Laboratory of Addictive Diseases, said of methadone: "It's a boring drug."[5] The high from taking a drug is determined in part by how much is taken but also by how rapidly it gets to the brain. In general the medications used for detoxification have a slow onset of action and metabolize out of the body slowly. These medications do have value in the illicit market for the same reasons that physicians prescribe them: to prevent the symptoms of withdrawal.

While medications to treat acute overdose and withdrawal are important and even lifesaving, these processes have a minimal effect on long-term remission from addiction. Medications that can help maintain remission show promise in affecting the long-term outcome of the diseases of addiction. The rest of this chapter will review the medications currently available for relapse prevention and describe some of the future directions of research in this area.

Medications for Preventing Relapse

The goal for medication use in relapse prevention is straightforward: to decrease the likelihood that the addicted individual will relapse to any drug use or at least to heavy drug use. Decreased use and preferably abstinence are prerequisites for creating a foundation on which a person can start to build her recovery. As mentioned in the previous chapter, stopping the use of drugs is huge, but is only the very beginning of remission. The hard work involves learning the personal and interpersonal skills needed to manage one's emotions, develop healthier relationships with family and friends, and begin to establish a new life. These life skills are the best defense against relapse, but in the meantime medications can help.

Medications used to decrease the likelihood of relapse act in several ways:

1. To replace the initial drug effects (agonist medication)
2. To decrease the craving that precedes relapse
3. To block the initial drug effects (antagonist medication)
4. To produce an unpleasant reaction when the drug of abuse is taken (aversive conditioning)

So far, there are approved medications only for alcohol, opioid, and nicotine addiction.

For many years, the only medication available to prevent relapse to alcohol use was disulfiram (Antabuse). Disulfiram blocks an enzyme in the metabolism of alcohol, leading to a buildup of the toxin acetaldehyde, which can cause flushing of the skin, nausea, vomiting, headache, and a dangerous drop in blood pressure if a person ingests alcohol. For a person committed to maintaining abstinence, disulfiram offers the following advantages:[6] first, taking the pill once daily confirms the decision not to drink that day; second, a person must wait to satisfy an impulse to drink for about five to seven days until disulfiram is out of his system, by which time the craving for alcohol will have dissipated; third, taking disulfiram daily expresses concretely the commitment to abstinence, whereas skipping doses or stopping the medication without first discussing it with one's physician suggests an impending relapse. Some of my patients have found disulfiram useful, but it is the fear of getting sick that supports their abstinence, rather than any pharmacological action of disulfiram that deters drinking. It should be no surprise that in randomized trials it performs no better than a placebo.[7]

Replacement medications have been in use since methadone was introduced in the mid-1960s.[8] The principle for using replacement medication is that the brain of an addicted person is no longer a normal brain and needs the drug or a replacement to diminish craving and prevent relapse to uncontrolled use of the initial drug. Whether the brain is able to return to more normal function or not depends on the severity of the addiction and the person's age. Younger brains are more plastic, which can make them more susceptible to the changes induced by drug use but also better able to repair the damage later. Currently there are accepted replacement medications for nicotine as well as the opioids.

Methadone for opioid dependence is available only in federally licensed methadone maintenance clinics. As a full agonist, methadone saturates the brain's *mu* opiate receptors. Its onset of action is slow, and it requires dosing once every twenty-four hours. (In contrast, when methadone is used for pain relief, it must be dosed every eight hours.) As the methadone level rises, the drug eliminates all symptoms of withdrawal. However, methadone abolishes craving only at significantly higher doses. Since all the opiate receptors are filled with methadone, any illicit opioid taken in addition to methadone has no binding site at which to produce its high. At the correct dose, methadone allows someone to function normally while resuming or beginning a more productive adult life.

The methadone clinic license, approved jointly by the Drug Enforcement Administration of the Department of Justice and the Food and Drug Administration (FDA) of the Department of Health and Human Services and regulated by the Substance Abuse and Mental Health Administration (SAMSHA) of the Department of Health and Human Services, specifies that individual and group counseling must be available to clinic clients so that appropriate psychosocial care is available. Clients whose urine drug screens have been negative for any illicit substances for several months may take home sufficient methadone for two up to six days rather than attend the clinic daily. Until 2003 and the advent of buprenorphine for opioid addiction, methadone was the only long-term medication consistently available to treat opioid addiction.

Buprenorphine is a partial agonist medication. Like methadone, which fills and activates a *mu* receptor site completely, buprenorphine blocks the *mu* receptor site and partially activates it, so that there are fewer effects of sedation and less risk of overdose. Buprenorphine also has a high affinity for these receptor sites and cannot be displaced by an illicit opioid (full agonist) taken in addition to buprenorphine. Like methadone, buprenorphine has a long half-life and can be taken once daily. Buprenorphine is absorbed through the membranes under the tongue and is not active if swallowed. To prevent diversion to injection drug use, most FDA-approved buprenorphine formulations are combined with the opiate antagonist naloxone, which is minimally absorbed sublingually. Its only purpose is to prevent the diversion of buprenorphine to intravenous use, by potentially precipitating severe and unpleasant withdrawal symptoms if injected.

Both buprenorphine and methadone at appropriate doses quell the intense craving for opioids that leads to relapse. While an average dose of sixty milligrams of methadone can prevent withdrawal symptoms, usually doses over one hundred milligrams are required to decrease craving, a major precipitant of relapse. Some patients on buprenorphine also require higher doses to reduce craving.

Both buprenorphine (without naloxone) and methadone are available for use by pregnant women. Use of methadone during pregnancy, instead of injecting drugs, is associated with better prenatal care and higher birth weights.[9] Because infants born to mothers on methadone or buprenorphine have these drugs in their system, the newborn must be detoxified after birth. The neonatal abstinence syndrome refers to the few days immediately after birth when the infant is abruptly cut off from the opioid in his mother's blood. This syndrome is treated like other withdrawal syndromes with reintoxication of the infant and then gradual taper of medication over the next several days. Although these babies are more irritable and startle more easily, current research does not show any evidence that these children do poorly cognitively and emotionally as they grow older.[10]

How long should patients stay on opioid replacement therapy? Is the goal eventual weaning off replacement therapy or maintenance for years? These questions miss the point. The goal of treatment is to help the patient optimize his functioning; for many, that will mean lifetime maintenance on these medications; for others, there is the possibility of eventually tapering off the replacement medication. But the data are not encouraging. For people on methadone maintenance who taper slowly off methadone over three to six months, the relapse rate approaches two-thirds.[11] Among all patients leaving methadone maintenance, the relapse rate is over 90 percent.[12] Yet this is typical of chronic diseases. Among hypertensive patients, for example, close to 100 percent would have high blood pressure readings if they stopped their blood pressure medications. Unless someone with hypertension is able to make drastic changes in lifestyle, he will need medication for the rest of his life. These maintenance medications, whether for addiction or hypertension, can control but not cure the underlying disease.

Methadone and buprenorphine are highly regulated because of concern that they will be diverted for illicit use. At the other end of the spectrum is nicotine replacement therapy, available to any adult over the counter. The circumstances are different, but the principles are the same.

Nicotine replacement therapy has been approved for detoxification from nicotine in tobacco. The slow-acting form of nicotine replacement, the transdermal patch, mitigates the withdrawal symptoms (headache, irritability, anxiety) that are potent triggers for relapse, but it does not address the acute craving for a cigarette. More rapid-acting forms of nicotine replacement, in the form of gum, lozenge, or nasal spray, can provide a more immediate boost of nicotine levels to ameliorate the craving sensations.

For those people who continue to relapse to tobacco abuse, long-term maintenance on nicotine replacement has seemed a reasonable option, and in April 2013, the FDA approved changes in labeling of nicotine replacement products to include long-term use.[13] Further, nicotine seems to have some positive effects for people with chronic mental illness,[14] a group that might benefit from long-term nicotine replacement to decrease their high risk for the cardiovascular consequences of cigarette smoking.[15]

Since one of the principles of replacement therapy is to find a cross-reacting drug that is longer acting with slower onset, there should be plenty of choices for alcohol addiction. The benzodiazepines act at the same neuroreceptors as alcohol, and several medications in this class have slow onset of action and long duration. Ironically, there is considerable hesitation in the addictions field to use these medications for alcohol addiction because of concern about addiction to the benzodiazepine and the additive sedating effects of combining a benzodiazepine and alcohol.

The decision to take a replacement medication involves a complicated calculus. These medications clearly prevent withdrawal syndromes and decrease craving as long as they are taken regularly. But there are the side effects of becoming physically dependent on the replacement medication or, more concerning, developing craving for the replacement medication itself. If the patient runs out of medication, there are the consequences of an unpleasant withdrawal syndrome. Isn't there a better way to manage craving without becoming dependent on another drug?

For the last two decades, research has focused on how to interrupt craving for different drugs. Craving is mediated through a subset of neurobiological pathways, mostly the *mu* opiate receptor. Naltrexone, the oral form of naloxone, is a complete antagonist at the *mu* receptor and decreases alcohol craving and use as measured by time to the first drink and to the first heavy drinking day.[16] It is available as a daily oral medication or a monthly depot injection. Acamprosate is another oral medication that decreases craving but through a different pathway. Although European studies have shown its effectiveness,[17] recent U.S. research indicates that naltrexone is more effective than acamprosate.[18]

Two medications, bupropion and varenicline, are approved to decrease craving for nicotine among tobacco users. Varenicline, much like buprenorphine at the *mu* opioid receptors, has both pro-nicotine and anti-nicotine effects at the nicotine receptors. These effects both moderate some withdrawal symptoms and decrease craving, but varenicline has potentially serious side effects of depression or heart problems. Bupropion, first marketed as an antidepressant, was found to decrease smoking in depressed individuals. Its exact mechanism in nicotine addiction is unclear, as it affects several neurotransmitter systems.[19] Combination therapy using both nicotine replacement and varenicline has resulted in about a 20 percent quit rate after six months.[20]

As scientists develop a more sophisticated understanding of the neurobiology of addiction, there will be new targets for intervention to interrupt the cycles of addiction. Several antiseizure medications appear to be effective in decreasing relapse to alcohol use.[21] Topiramate is a good example. It affects the neuroreceptors involved in alcohol intoxication and dependence in exactly the opposite way that alcohol acts on these receptors. Compared to subjects treated with placebo, those treated with topiramate had a decreased percentage of heavy drinking days.[22]

The challenge remains that the neural pathways involved in drug addiction are basic, fundamental pathways necessary for healthy brain function. Tampering with them may have unintended consequences. The medications that do exist have somewhat limited effects on the overall course of a person's addiction. Over the next decade, I expect that there will be a proliferation of medications to treat addiction. Hopefully, they will relieve the very real suffering of addiction, but the work of effectively managing this chronic illness will still require psychological and behavioral changes that only the patient can make.

EPILOGUE

People say you should write the introduction and the conclusion before you write the book. The introduction I can understand, but writing a book takes you on a journey, and you may end up in an unexpected place. This is as true of my patients' journeys of addiction as it is of my own life. My professional and personal lives have fueled my passion to help others understand this chronic illness and the lives of those who experience it.

The very complex disease of addiction affects basic brain functioning. We all rely on habits to provide the patterns of daily life. These helpful structures usually reflect the ordering of priorities and values. We get up in the morning, brush our teeth, get dressed, and go off to work without much forethought. The ways we interact with family and friends, the ways we think about current events are habits of the mind. We learn to subsume some of our basic desires under the lattice of these habits.

With addiction, the tables are turned. Basic reward pathways are co-opted by drugs or certain behaviors, such as compulsive gambling. The compulsion to use drugs overwhelms normal behaviors, creating habitual activities dedicated to the procurement and use of the drug. These compulsive activities dictate changes in brain function and structure that make these behaviors difficult to disrupt and extinguish. This is the work of a diseased brain. Martha's request to her psychiatrist to prescribe the same anxiety medication that had triggered several long relapses told me how severe her addiction is. Her decision to taper off this medication tells me she has a fighting chance, but the prognosis of her addictions is uncertain.

Writing this book has helped me appreciate how my patients have become addicted. The insidious interplay of genetic and environmental factors creates vulnerabilities that are difficult to overcome. People in any socioeconomic class can succumb to the genetic vulnerabilities that lead to addiction, but the environmental vulnerabilities more often affect those in poverty and with few social resources. So many of my addicted patients have family histories of addiction and mental illness. So many suffered as children from the absence of a consistent and loving environment, because their parents were struggling with their own addiction and mental health issues.

Linda, whose parents suffered from addiction and mental illness, continues to care for her two teenage daughters and attend community college. She has not relapsed to opiate use in over five years and has decreased her smoking. Her ever-present depression is manageable on a new medication. She does not attend AA or NA, but she is developing connections with sober adults, fellow parents from her daughters' swimming and basketball teams. She can now acknowledge her own pride in what she has accomplished. Her prognosis is very good.

Problems with drug use often occur in a vacuum of parental oversight. Without his mother's love and protection, Larry found opiates relieved the pain of her death. His early years of addiction were fraught with impulsive behaviors and poor judgment as he tried to prevent his grief and sadness from overwhelming him. Eight years later, he continues to struggle. He has had one or two brief lapses in the last year and has completed a four-week intensive outpatient program. Because of his anxiety, he has not completed training to be an auto mechanic, but he is thinking more about his future. He is still homeless, staying with friends, but he has taken control of and responsibility for his own life. Larry is moving forward slowly, but his trauma and depression dog his steps. His prognosis for a stable recovery and a more satisfying life is uncertain, but he has surprised me before.

Within the all-consuming nature of addiction lie the seeds of its demise. The price it exacts in loss of self-respect, fractured relationships with family and friends, financial ruin, and poverty of spirit turns people against their addiction even as it continues to consume them. "I don't want to use; I don't even like using . . . and yet, I just did," puzzles Bill, coming back after a relapse. Addiction treatment exploits this inner contradiction. In understanding his ambivalence, Bill articulated what he did and did not like about using drugs. His treatment plan had to address both the needs that the drug satisfied and the chaos in his personal and emotional life. He had to overcome the manipulative behavior and dishonesty that characterize addicted behavior.

After each relapse to injecting opiates, Bill had found his way to abstinence. He sought treatment at local detoxification centers, month-long rehabilitation programs, and out-of-state halfway houses. Each time he returned more thoughtful about his addiction and more committed to recovery; each time, boredom, the lack of affordable addictions treatment, and the frustration of not finding work precipitated another relapse. One day at a time over the last five years, he has been able to engage in AA long enough to get a sponsor and to complete a vocational program. When he did get a job, as a long-distance truck driver, he faced a dilemma. He needed the income, but he no longer had the frequent support of his AA group and was offered more drugs on the road than when at home. He knows his recovery is at risk. He recently quit long-distance driving and has found a job closer to home. In his words, "My recovery has to come first."

Initially, his immaturity, self-loathing, and the severity of his addiction made me pessimistic about his recovery. I was wrong. His job driving a delivery truck for a big company is secure and has good benefits. With his commitment to the principles of AA and to his AA friends, he has created his community. As he told me recently, his anxiety and depression are much better and no longer require medication. His encompassing self-hatred as he began treatment has matured into an understanding that his intense shame and guilt from fifteen years of addiction still block his progress. I expect he may use drugs once or twice in the future when overwhelmed by negative feelings or unforeseen challenges, but I am no longer very worried. His prognosis is excellent.

I am humbled by how hard these people work to keep themselves afloat and by how slow and torturous this process of recovery can be. Even Russell and Jackie, after more than fifteen years of recovery, still relied on regular involvement with AA for support until their untimely addiction-related deaths.

I have been a witness to their pain, but have I helped more than that? For some, I have perhaps been a catalyst in their struggles to move forward. With others, I have watched years of suffering with transient improvements. Perhaps catalyst is the wrong word, for it implies that I have positively affected their course of treatment without being changed myself. Nothing could be further from the truth. I have been moved to tears and to anger by their behavior. I have cried with them and celebrated tiny successes. I have felt completely proud of their efforts and hopelessly duped by some of their lies. With the former, I experience a profound partnership with the patient. She and I are allied against the devastating forces of addiction. Together we strategize how to tame this overwhelming disease.

Delia has had a difficult few years. Every four to six months, her recovery has been punctuated by another crisis—the death of a close friend, theft of her Social Security disability checks, friction with her family, and an abusive relationship. Her most recent relapse to cocaine and amphetamines precipitated severe agitation, anxiety, and a paranoid psychosis that persisted for several months. She received some emergency psychiatric treatment, pulled herself back into sobriety, and continued using Suboxone to prevent a relapse to opiates. She has not used any drugs, except nicotine, in the past three months, but she is still too disorganized and depressed to find support in NA meetings or commit to regular counseling. She will lose her housing next month and has only her dysfunctional family to fall back on. As her primary care physician, I am currently providing her medical, addictions, and psychiatric care. She needs much more help than I can offer. Without it, her prognosis is guarded.

Many of my patients with chronic illnesses are not interested in fancy medical technologies or a prescription for the newest drug to treat their illness; they just want me to be there. The most helpful intervention is simply to bear witness, to sit in the presence of someone else's pain and not flinch. When the pain is expressed as lies and manipulations, I have learned to hear the pathetic sadness behind the lies. My initial sense of anger is irrelevant. These manipulations are not about me, but about the patient's inability to be honest and direct with herself. She is still in the throes of her addiction. If she can risk making a connection with me, I may be able to help her. During the mid-twentieth century, Dr. Michael Balint, a Hungarian general practitioner and psychoanalyst best known for his studies on the psychological implications of patient-doctor relationships in general practice (primary care), wrote "certainly not for the first time in history" his work revealed "that by far the most frequently used drug in general practice is *the doctor himself*" (original emphasis).[1] Despite all the medical advances in the last seventy-five years, that comment is still true in primary care practice.

These patients, suffering from addiction or other devastating chronic illnesses, have enriched my life with their determination, perseverance, humor, and humility. They have taught me about the burdens of pain, disappointment, and failure, and the strengths needed to survive, endure, and succeed. An unexpected gift has touched me deeply. Their courage and resilience, despite formidable odds, have given me the courage to stand tall in my own shoes. Like my addicted patients, my own chronic illness has its genetic and environmental roots. Starting in adolescence, depression disrupted my education and medical training, confirmed my own sense of failure, and introduced me to the long shadow of stigma. Unlike many of my patients with chronic illnesses, I received intensive treatment when I needed it and long-term follow-up when I needed that. I have had my relapses and remissions. Medication and support have helped to keep my illness manageable for many years. I know that I am very fortunate. Now, my envious reaction as an unhappy, stressed medical student attending her first AA meeting makes sense to me. Surrounded by AA members living with a chronic, stigmatized illness, I had experienced communal feelings of gratitude and hope way beyond my grasp. Decades later, working with my patients who fight to control their addictions and build better lives, I can sense with more resonance than they realize their early glimmers of gratitude and hope.

Despite my patients' difficulties in getting the help they need, I am cautiously optimistic. Our scientific understanding of addiction is improving rapidly, which should lead to better behavioral treatments and new medications. A growing number of health professionals have received training in addictions. Screening and early treatment for drug problems, as well as ongoing management of them, have been extended into the primary care community. We are making progress, but too slowly.

Where, one might ask, is the urgency? To which I would reply: Delia is a few weeks away from homelessness and likely her next relapse. Bill and Martha understand that another relapse might kill them. Thousands of young people are dying annually from prescription opioid overdoses. The carnage on our highways continues. My patients are battling to maintain their recoveries despite a paucity of resources. Many more want treatment but cannot get it. Several times a week I receive e-mails through a national website from patients looking for office-based opiate treatment. I wish that I could accommodate them.

Meanwhile our government still prefers to approach addiction as a criminal justice problem. More government funding goes to interrupt the big business of the drug trade or to incarcerate low-level offenders than to prevention and treatment combined. Knowledge of this treatable brain disease has the power to overcome stigma and to help us set more humane policies and laws. We need to change our priorities to emphasize prevention and treatment. We owe it to our children and siblings, our friends and neighbors who wrestle with this disease.

My hope is that this book will help move the conversation toward understanding, compassion, and, above all, action.

NOTES

INTRODUCTION

1. Russell Brazil (1949–2007), with permission from his wife, Christine Brazil.

2. Melonie Heron, "Deaths: Leading Causes 2009," ed. National Center for Vital Statistics (Hyattsville, MD: National Center for Health Statistics, 2012).

3. "Addiction Science: From Molecules to Managed Care," National Institute on Drug Abuse, accessed May 12, 2013, www.drugabuse.gov.

4. Ibid.; "Vital Signs: Overdoses of Prescription Opioid Pain Relievers—United States, 1998–2008," *Morbidity and Mortality Weekly Report* 60, no. 43 (2011), accessed May 12, 2013, www.cdc.gov.

5. "Impaired Driving: Get the Facts," Centers for Disease Control and Prevention, accessed May 12, 2013, www.cdc.gov.

6. "Average for U. S. 2001–2005—Years of Potential Life Lost Due to Excessive Alcohol Use," Centers for Disease Control and Prevention, accessed May 12, 2013, apps.nccd.cdc.gov.

7. T. Miller and D. Hendrie, "Substance Abuse Prevention Dollars and Cents: A Cost-Benefit Analysis," ed. Substance Abuse and Mental Health Services Administration, Center for Substance Abuse Prevention (Rockville, MD: U.S. Department of Health and Human Services, 2008).

8. S. L. West and K. K. O'Neal, "Project D.A.R.E. Outcome Effectiveness Revisited," *American Journal of Public Health* 94, no. 6 (2004).

9. World Health Organization, "The Tenth Revision of the International Classification of Diseases and Health Problems (ICD-10)," accessed Jun 5, 2006, www.who.int.

10. J. Harry Isaacson et al., "A National Survey of Training in Substance Use Disorders in Residency Programs," *Journal of Studies on Alcohol and Drugs* 61, no. 6 (2000); Norman S. Miller et al., "Why Physicians Are Unprepared to Treat Patients Who Have Alcohol- and Drug-Related Disorders," *Academic Medicine* 76, no. 5 (2001).

11. Patrick Griswold and Hillary Jacobs, *Waking Up: A Film about Opiate Addiction and Recovery* (funded by the Bonney Family Foundation and the Society for the Arts in Healthcare [RWJ], 2006).

12. Francis Weld Peabody, *Doctor and Patient* (New York: MacMillan Company, 1930), 52.

ONE. LEARNING TO USE

1. Koren Zailckas, *Smashed: Story of a Drunken Girlhood*, paperback ed. (New York: Penguin Group, 2006).

2. Ibid., 91–96.

3. Mark D. Merlin, *On the Trail of the Ancient Opium Poppy* (Cranbury, NJ: Associated University Press, 1984), chap. 5, passim.

4. Ibid., chap. 6, passim.

5. Martin Booth, *Opium: A History* (London: Simon & Schuster, 1996), 105–6.

6. Ibid., 112–14.

7. E. Jean Matteson Langdon, "Shamanism and Anthropology," in *Portals of Power: Shamanism in South America*, ed. E. Jean Matteson Langdon and Gerhard Baer (Albuquerque: University of New Mexico Press, 1992), 17.

8. E. Jean Matteson Langdon, "Dau: Shamanic Power in Siona Religion," in *Portals of Power*, ed. E. Jean Matteson Langdon and Gerhard Baer (Albuquerque: University of New Mexico Press, 1992), 141.

9. Samuel Z. Klausner and Edward F. Foulks, *Eskimo Capitalists: Oil, Politics, and Alcohol* (Totowa, N.J.: Allenheld, Osmun & Co., 1982); Michael Pollan, *The Botany of Desire* (New York: Random House, 2001).

10. Pollan, *The Botany of Desire*, 217.

11. Matthew, "The Gospel According to Matthew," in *The New Testament of Our Lord and Savior Jesus Christ* (New York: The World Publishing Company, 1962).

12. *The Qur'an: A Modern English Version*, trans. Majid Fakhry, paperback ed. (Reading, UK: Garnet Publishing, 1997). sura 5, 90, and sura 47, 16.

13. Booth, *Opium*, 81.

14. Zailckas, *Smashed*, 23.

15. Donald Dale Jackson, *Gold Dust: The California Gold Rush and the Forty-Niners* (London: George Allen & Unwin, 1980), 292; J. S. Holliday, *Rush for Riches: Gold Fever and the Making of California* (San Francisco: University of California Press, 1999), 214.

16. V. Casikar et al., "Does Chewing Coca Leaves Influence Physiology at High Altitude?" *Indian Journal of Clinical Biochemistry* 25, no. 3 (2010).

17. William Stewart, *The Surgeon General's Report on Smoking: 1968 Supplement to Public Health Service Publication 1696*, ed. U.S. Department of Health (U.S. Printing Office, 1968).

18. Martin Torgoff, *Can't Find My Way Home* (New York: Simon & Schuster, 2004), 104.

19. Ibid., 201.

20. Substance Abuse and Mental Health Services Administration, "Results from the 2011 National Survey on Drug Use and Health: Summary of National Findings," NSDUH Series H-44, HHS Publication No. (SMA) 12-4713 (Rockville, MD: Substance Abuse and Mental Health Services Administration, 2012).

21. Ibid.

22. L. D. Johnston et al., "Monitoring the Future National Results on Drug Use: 2012 Overview; Key Findings on Adolescent Drug Use" (Ann Arbor, MI: Institute for Social Research, University of Michigan, 2013).

23. William A. Vega et al., "Prevalence and Age of Onset for Drug Use in Seven International Sites: Results from the International Consortium of Psychiatric Epidemiology," *Drug and Alcohol Dependence* 68, no. 3 (2002).

24. Eleni Houghton and Ann M. Roche, eds., *Learning about Drinking*, International Center for Alcohol Policies Series on Alcohol and Society (Philadelphia: Taylor & Francis, 2001); L. Degenhardt et al., "Evaluating the Drug Use 'Gateway' Theory Using Cross-National Data: Consistency and Associations of the Order of Initiation of Drug Use among Participants in the WHO World Mental Health Surveys," *Drug and Alcohol Dependence* 108, no. 1–2 (2010).

25. Carol D. Frary, Rachel K. Johnson, and Min Qi Wang, "Food Sources and Intakes of Caffeine in the Diets of Persons in the United States," *Journal of the American Dietetic Association* 105, no. 1 (2005).

26. All public use is proscribed, but approximately half of the states have statutes that permit use of alcohol at home in the presence of family members.

27. Robert Scragg, Murray Laugesen, and Elizabeth Robinson, "Parental Smoking and Related Behaviours Influence Adolescent Tobacco Smoking: Results from the 2001 New Zealand National Survey of 4th Form Students," *New Zealand Medical Journal* 116, no. 1187 (2003).

28. George E. Vaillant, *The Natural History of Alcoholism Revisited* (Cambridge, MA: Harvard University Press, 1995; repr., 2000); Michael A. Collins et al., "Alcohol in Moderation, Cardioprotection, and Neuroprotection: Epidemiological Considerations and Mechanistic Studies," *Alcoholism: Clinical and Experimental Research* 33, no. 2 (2009): 139–41.

29. L. Alan Sroufe et al., *The Development of the Person: The Minnesota Study of Risk and Adaptation from Birth to Adulthood* (New York: Guildford Press, 2005).

30. Michelle M. Englund et al., "The Developmental Significance of Late Adolescent Substance Use for Early Adult Functioning," *Developmental Psychology* (Oct 1, 2012). Adolescents were assigned to one of four groups according to frequency and consequences of drug use: Abstainers—never used alcohol or other drugs; Experimenters—used alcohol or marijuana with low frequency, but no other illicit drugs; At Risk users—used alcohol, marijuana, and/or other illicit drugs and experienced some difficulty functioning due to drugs but did not meet criteria for a substance use disorder; Abusers—met criteria for a substance use disorder with a pattern of repeated problems in at least two areas of functioning.

31. B. J. Casey et al., "Imaging the Developing Brain: What Have We Learned about Cognitive Development?" *Trends in Cognitive Sciences* 9, no. 3 (2005).

32. Nitin Gogtay et al., "Dynamic Mapping of Human Cortical Development during Childhood through Early Adulthood," *Proceedings of the National Academy of Sciences of the United States of America* 101, no. 21 (2004).

33. Elizabeth R. Sowell et al., "Mapping Continued Brain Growth and Gray Matter Density Reduction in Dorsal Frontal Cortex: Inverse Relationships during Postadolescent Brain Maturation," *Journal of Neuroscience* 21, no. 22 (2001).

34. Gogtay et al., "Dynamic Mapping."

35. Leah H. Somerville and B. J. Casey, "Developmental Neurobiology of Cognitive Control and Motivational Systems," *Current Opinion in Neurobiology* 20, no. 2 (2010).

36. Elizabeth R. Sowell, Paul M. Thompson, and Arthur W. Toga, "Mapping Changes in the Human Cortex throughout the Span of Life," *Neuroscientist* 10, no. 4 (2004).

37. B. J. Casey and Rebecca M. Jones, "Neurobiology of the Adolescent Brain and Behavior: Implications for Substance Use Disorders," *Journal of the American Academy of Child & Adolescent Psychiatry* 49, no. 12 (2010).

38. Susan Barron et al., "Adolescent Vulnerabilities to Chronic Alcohol or Nicotine Exposure: Findings from Rodent Models," *Alcoholism: Clinical and Experimental Research* 29, no. 9 (2005); Robert F. Smith, "Animal Models of Periadolescent Substance Abuse," *Neurotoxicology and Teratology* 25, no. 3 (2003).

39. Jennifer A. Trauth et al., "Adolescent Nicotine Exposure Produces Immediate and Long-Term Changes in CNS Noradrenergic and Dopaminergic Function," *Brain Research* 892, no. 2 (2001).

40. Conversation between H. Scott Swartzwelder, Ph.D., Professor of Psychiatry at Duke University, and the author on Aug 3, 2006.

41. Smith, "Animal Models."

42. Peter M. Monti et al., "Adolescence: Booze, Brains, and Behavior," *Alcoholism: Clinical and Experimental Research* 29, no. 2 (2005); Barron et al., "Adolescent Vulnerabilities."

43. Fulton T. Crews et al., "Neurogenesis in Adolescent Brains Is Potently Inhibited by Ethanol," *Neuroscience* 137 (2006); Jennifer A. Obernier et al., "Cognitive Deficits and CNS Damage after a 4-Day Binge Ethanol Exposure in Rats," *Pharmacology Biochemistry and Behavior* 72, no. 3 (2002).

44. Crews et al., "Neurogenesis in Adolescent Brains."

45. Obernier et al., "Cognitive Deficits."

46. Kimberly Nixon and Fulton T. Crews, "Binge Ethanol Exposure Decreases Neurogenesis in Adult Rat Hippocampus," *Journal of Neurochemistry* 83, no. 5 (2002); Jennifer A. Obernier, T. W. Bouldin, and F. T. Crews, "Binge Ethanol Exposure in Adult Rats Causes Necrotic Cell Death," *Alcoholism: Clinical and Experimental Research* 26, no. 4 (2002).

47. Fulton T. Crews et al., "Binge Ethanol Consumption Causes Differential Brain Damage in Young Adolescent Rats Compared with Adult Rats," *Alcoholism: Clinical and Experimental Research* 24, no. 11 (2000).

48. Craig J. Slawecki et al., "Periadolescent Alcohol Exposure Has Lasting Effects on Adult Neurophysiological Function in Rats," *Developmental Brain Research* 128, no. 1 (2001); G. K. Pyapali et al., "Age and Dose-Dependent Effects of Ethanol on the Induction of Hippocampal Long-Term Potentiation," *Alcohol* 19 no. 2 (1999).

49. Helena J. V. Rutherford, Linda C. Mayes, and Marc N. Potenza, "Neurobiology of Adolescent Substance Use Disorders: Implications for Prevention and Treatment," *Child and Adolescent Psychiatric Clinics of North America* 19, no. 3 (2010).

50. H. S. Swartzwelder et al., "Developmental Differences in the Acquisition of Tolerance to Ethanol," *Alcohol* 15, no. 4 (1998). The rats were treated with 4 mg/kg of alcohol twice daily for three to seven days. For a 60 kg woman, the equivalent dose would be 480 mg alcohol. An "average" drink contains between 12 and 15 grams of pure alcohol. The total consumption would be 32 to 40 drinks daily.

51. S. K. Acheson, E. L. Ross, and H. S. Swartzwelder, "Age-Independent and

Dose-Response Effects of Ethanol on Spatial Memory in Rats," *Alcohol* 23, no. 3 (2001).

52. Elena I. Varlinskaya and Linda P. Spear, "Differences in the Social Consequences of Ethanol Emerge during the Course of Adolescence in Rats: Social Facilitation, Social Inhibition, and Anxiolysis," *Developmental Psychobiology* 48, no. 2 (2006).

53. Aaron M. White et al., "Differential Effects of Ethanol on Motor Coordination in Adolescent and Adult Rats," *Pharmacology Biochemistry and Behavior* 73, no. 3 (2002); Swartzwelder et al., "Developmental Differences"; Young May Cha et al., "Sedative and GABAergic Effects of Ethanol on Male and Female Rats," *Alcoholism: Clinical and Experimental Research* 30, no. 1 (2006).; Patrick J. Little et al., "Differential Effects of Ethanol in Adolescent and Adult Rats," *Alcoholism: Clinical and Experimental Research* 20, no. 8 (1996).

54. Elena I. Varlinskaya and Linda P. Spear, "Acute Ethanol Withdrawal (Hangover) and Social Behavior in Adolescent and Adult Male and Female Sprague-Dawley Rats," *Alcoholism: Clinical and Experimental Research* 28, no. 1 (2004).

55. Aaron M. White and H. Scott Swartzwelder, "Age-Related Effects of Alcohol on Memory and Memory-Related Brain Function in Adolescents and Adults," *Recent Developments in Alcoholism* 17 (2005).

56. Alecia D. Schweinsburg, Bonnie J. Nagel, and Susan F. Tapert, "FMRI Reveals Alteration of Spatial Working Memory Networks across Adolescence," *Journal of the International Neuropsychological Society* 11, no. 5 (2005).

57. Barbara J. Markwiese et al., "Differential Effects of Ethanol on Memory in Adolescent and Adult Rats," *Alcoholism: Clinical and Experimental Research* 22, no. 2 (1998).

58. Denise Siciliano and Robert F. Smith, "Periadolescent Alcohol Alters Adult Behavioral Characteristics in the Rat," *Physiology and Behavior* 74 (2001).

59. Tamara L. Doremus et al., "Factors Influencing Elevated Ethanol Consumption in Adolescent Relative to Adult Rats," *Alcoholism: Clinical and Experimental Research* 29, no. 10 (2005).

60. Swartzwelder et al., "Developmental Differences."

61. Moriah N. Strong et al., "'Binge' Drinking Experience in Adolescent Mice Shows Sex Differences and Elevated Ethanol Intake in Adulthood," *Hormones and Behavior* 58, no. 1 (2010).

62. Jennifer A. Trauth et al., "Adolescent Nicotine Exposure Causes Persistent Upregulation of Nicotinic Cholinergic Receptors in Rat Brain Regions," *Brain Research* 851, no. 1–2 (1999).

63. A. R. Zavala et al., "Cocaine-Induced Behavioral Sensitization in the Young Rat," *Psychopharmacology (Berl)* 151, no. 2–3 (2000).

64. Theodore A. Slotkin and Frederic J. Seidler, "Nicotine Exposure in Adolescence Alters the Response of Serotonin Systems to Nicotine Administered Subsequently in Adulthood," *Developmental Neuroscience* 31, no. 1–2 (2009).

65. Smith, "Animal Models."

66. Siciliano and Smith, "Periadolescent Alcohol."

67. Ibid.

68. Aaron M. White et al., "Binge Pattern Ethanol Exposure in Adolescent and

Adult Rats: Differential Impact on Subsequent Responsiveness to Ethanol," *Alcoholism: Clinical and Experimental Research* 24, no. 8 (2000).

69. E. D. Levin, "Persisting Effects of Chronic Adolescent Nicotine Administration on Radial-Arm Maze Learning and Response to Nicotine Challenges," *Neurotoxicology and Teratology* 21 (1999); Robert F. Smith, C. N. Medici, and D. K. Raap, "Enduring Behavioral Effects of Weaning-through-Puberty Cocaine Dosing in the Rat," *Psychobiology* 27 (1999).

70. Smith, "Animal Models."

71. Marco Pistis et al., "Adolescent Exposure to Cannabinoids Induces Long-Lasting Changes in the Response to Drugs of Abuse of Rat Midbrain Dopamine Neurons," *Biological Psychiatry* 56, no. 2 (2004).

72. Sroufe et al., *The Development of the Person.*

73. Ibid., ix.

74. Ibid., x.

75. Ibid., 173.

76. Ibid., 66.

77. Ibid., 184. Early experience included maternal sensitivity and cooperation (infant aged 6 months), attachment security (12–18 months), toddler experience (24 months), and early childhood experience (42 months).

78. Gerard M. Schippers et al., "Acquiring the Competence to Drink Responsibly," in *Learning about Drinking,* ed. Eleni Houghton and Ann M. Roche, International Center for Alcohol Policies Series on Alcohol and Society (Philadelphia: Taylor & Francis, 2001), 42; Jonathan Shedler and Jack Block, "Adolescent Drug Use and Psychological Health: A Longitudinal Inquiry," *American Psychologist* 45, no. 5 (1990).

79. Vaillant, *The Natural History of Alcoholism Revisited,* 131, 144.

80. Shedler and Block, "Adolescent Drug Use."

81. Ibid.

82. Ibid., 194, 196.

83. J. Siebenbruner et al., "Developmental Antecedents of Late Adolescence Substance Use Patterns," *Development and Psychopathology* 18, no. 2 (2006).

84. See above, note 30, for definitions of the four groups of adolescents (abstainers, experimenters, at-risk users, and abusers).

85. Siebenbruner et al., "Developmental Antecedents"; personal communication, Michelle Englund, Ph.D., Research Associate, Institute of Child Development, University of Minnesota and the Center for Analysis of Pathways from childhood to Adulthood, Aug 8, 2006.

86. Michelle M. Englund et al., "Childhood and Adolescent Predictors of Heavy Drinking and Alcohol Use Disorders in Early Adulthood: A Longitudinal Developmental Analysis," *Addiction* 103, suppl 1 (2008).

87. Sroufe et al., *The Development of the Person.*

88. Englund et al., "Childhood and Adolescent Predictors."

89. Michelle Englund, unpublished data (Institute of Child Development, University of Minnesota and the Center for Analysis of Pathways from Childhood to Adulthood, 2006).

90. Substance Abuse and Mental Health Services Administration, "Results from the 2011 National Survey."

91. National Institute on Alcohol Abuse and Alcoholism, "A Clinician's Guide to Alcohol Use" (National Institutes of Health, 2004).

TWO. SCIENCE OF ADDICTION

1. American Psychiatric Association, *Diagnostic and Statistical Manual of Mental Disorders*, 4th ed., text rev (DSM-IV-TR) (Washington, DC: American Psychiatric Association, 2000).

2. George E. Vaillant, *The Natural History of Alcoholism: Causes, Patterns, and Paths to Recovery* (Cambridge, MA: Harvard University Press, 1983), 59–64.

3. Benei Noaj, ed. *Alcoholics Anonymous Big Book: Special Edition Including New Personal Stories for the Year 2007* (AA Services, 2006), 12, 17, 30, 103.

4. Vaillant, *The Natural History of Alcoholism*; K. M. Fillmore, "Relationships between Specific Drinking Problems in Early Adulthood and Middle Age," *Journal of Studies on Alcohol* 36 (1975); R Jessor, "Problem-Behavior Theory, Psychosocial Development and Adolescent Problem Drinking," *British Journal of Addictions* 82 (1987).

5. Neil Levy, ed., *Addiction and Self-Control: Perspectives from Philosophy, Psychology, and Neuroscience* (New York, NY: Oxford University Press, 2013).

6. Nora D. Volkow et al., "Unbalanced Neuronal Circuits in Addiction," *Current Opinion in Neurobiology* 23, no. 4 (2013).

7. Ann E. Kelley and Kent C. Berridge, "The Neuroscience of Natural Rewards: Relevance to Addictive Drugs," *Journal of Neuroscience* 22, no. 9 (2002).

8. T. W. Robbins and B. J. Everitt, "Drug Addiction: Bad Habits Add Up," *Nature* 398, no. 6728 (1999).

9. Steven E. Hyman, Robert C. Malenka, and Eric J. Nestler, "Neural Mechanisms of Addiction: The Role of Reward-Related Learning and Memory," *Annual Review of Neuroscience* 29 (2006).

10. B. J. Everitt and T. W. Robbins, "Neural Systems of Reinforcement for Drug Addiction: From Actions to Habits to Compulsion," *Nature Neuroscience* 8 (2005).

11. N. D. Volkow, Joanna S. Fowler, and Gene-Jack Wang, "The Addicted Human Brain Viewed in the Light of Imaging Studies: Brain Circuits and Treatment Strategies," *Neuropharmacology* 47 suppl 1 (2004).

12. Brian T. Miller and Mark D'Esposito, "Searching for 'the Top' in Top-Down Control," *Neuron* 48, no. 4 (2005).

13. Hyman, Malenka, and Nestler, "Neural Mechanisms of Addiction: The Role of Reward-Related Learning and Memory."

14. Volkow et al., "Unbalanced Neuronal Circuits."

15. Vincent P. Dole, Marie E. Nyswander, and Mary Jeanne Kreek, "Narcotic Blockade," *Archives of Internal Medicine* 118, no. 4 (1966).

16. Steven E. Hyman, "The Neurobiology of Addiction: Implications for Voluntary Control of Behavior," *American Journal of Bioethics* 7, no. 1 (2007); Robbins and Everitt, "Drug Addiction."

17. Wolfram Schultz, "Behavioral Theories and the Neurophysiology of Reward," *Annual Review of Psychology* 57 (2006).

18. Ibid.

19. Natalie C. Tronson and Jane R. Taylor, "Addiction: A Drug-Induced Disorder of Memory Reconsolidation," *Current Opinion in Neurobiology* 23, no. 4 (2013).

20. Kent C Berridge, "From Prediction Error to Incentive Salience: Mesolimbic Computation of Reward Motivation," *European Journal of Neuroscience* 35, no. 7 (2012).

21. Schultz, "Behavioral Theories."

22. Robbins and Everitt, "Drug Addiction."

23. Volkow, Fowler, and Wang, "The Addicted Human Brain."

24. Robbins and Everitt, "Drug Addiction."

25. Hyman, "The Neurobiology of Addiction."

26. Robbins and Everitt, "Drug Addiction"; Hyman, Malenka, and Nestler, "Neural mechanisms of Addiction"; George F. Koob, "The Neurobiology of Addiction: A Neuroadaptational View Relevant for Diagnosis," *Addiction* 101, suppl 1 (2006).

27. Steven E. Hyman, "Addiction: A Disease of Learning and Memory," *American Journal of Psychiatry* 162, no. 8 (2005).

28. George F. Koob and Michel Le Moal, "Plasticity of Reward Neurocircuitry and the 'Dark Side' of Drug addiction," *NaturenNeuroscience* 8, no. 11 (2005); Everitt and Robbins, "Neural Systems of Reinforcement"; Nora D. Volkow and Joanna S. Fowler, "Addiction, a Disease of Compulsion and Drive: Involvement of the Orbitofrontal Cortex," *Cerebral Cortex* 10 (2000).

29. Volkow et al., "Unbalanced Neuronal Circuits."

30. Lucinda Miner, "Neurobiology of Addiction," in *Clinical Teaching in Addiction Medicine: A Chief Resident Immersion Training (CRIT) Program* (Chatham, MA, 2006).

31. Volkow, Fowler, and Wang, "The Addicted Human Brain."

32. Rita Z. Goldstein and Nora D. Volkow, "Dysfunction of the Prefrontal Cortex in Addiction: Neuroimaging Findings and Clinical Implications," *Nature Reviews Neuroscience* 12, no. 11 (2011).

33. Rita Z. Goldstein and Nora D. Volkow, "Drug Addiction and Its Underlying Neurobiological Basis: Neuroimaging Evidence for the Involvement of the Frontal Cortex," *American Journal of Psychiatry* 159, no. 10 (2002).

34. Mark Walton and Nicholas Nasrallah, "Varieties of Valuation in the Normal and Addicted Brain: Legal and Policy Implications from a Neuroscience Perspective," in Neil Levy, ed., *Addiction and Self-Control: Perspectives from Philosophy, Psychology, and Neuroscience* (New York, NY: Oxford University Press, 2013).

35. Hyman, Malenka, and Nestler, "Neural Mechanisms of Addiction"; J. D. Berke and S. E. Hyman, "Addiction, Dopamine, and the Molecular Mechanisms of Memory," *Neuron* 25, no. 3 (2000).

36. Koob and Le Moal, "Plasticity of Reward Neurocircuitry."

37. George F. Koob and M. Le Moal, "Drug Abuse: Hedonic Homeostatic Dysregulation," *Science* 278, no. 5335 (1997).

38. George F Koob, "Negative Reinforcement in Drug Addiction: The Darkness Within," *Current Opinion in Neurobiology* (Apr 26, 2013).

39. T. E. Robinson and K. C. Berridge, "Addiction," *Annual Review of Psychology* 54 (2003).

40. Daniel M. Wegner, *The Illusion of Conscious Will* (Cambridge, MA: The MIT Press, 2002).

41. Bernhard Schlink, *The Reader,* trans. Carol Brown Janeway (New York: Pantheon Books, 1997), 21.

42. Substance Abuse and Mental Health Services Administration, "National Survey on Drug Use and Health [hereafter NSDUH]," Substance Abuse and Mental Health Services Administration (2012), accessed Aug 12, 2013, www.samhsa.gov /data/NSDUH.aspx. Substance Abuse and Mental Health Services Administration, "National Household Survey on Drug Abuse," ed. of Applied Services Office (1998).

43. Sroufe et al., *The Development of the Person*.

44. Jessor, "Problem-Behavior Theory"; W. McCord and J. McCord, *Origins of Alcoholism* (Stanford, CA: Stanford University Press, 1960).

45. Vaillant, *The Natural History of Alcoholism*; Vaillant, *The Natural History of Alcoholism Revisited*.

46. Vaillant, *Triumphs of Experience: The Men of the Harvard Grant Study* (Cambridge, MA: The Belknap Press of Harvard University Press, 2012).

47. Sheldon Glueck and Eleanor Glueck, *Delinquents and Nondelinquents in Perspective* (Cambridge, MA: Harvard University Press, 1968).

48. D. Cahalan and R. Room, "Problem Drinking among American Men Aged 21–59," *American Journal of Public Health* 62, no. 11 (1972).

49. American Psychiatric Association, *Diagnostic and Statistical Manual of Mental Disorders*, 5th ed. (DSM-5) (Arlington, VA; www.dsm5.org, accessed Jan 8, 2014).

50. L. D. Johnston et al., "Monitoring the Future National Results on Adolescent Drug Use: Overview of Key Findings, 2005" (National Institutes of Health, 2006); Substance Abuse and Mental Health Services Administration, "NSDUH"; Substance Abuse and Mental Health Services Administration, "National Household Survey on Drug Abuse," ed. Applied Services Office (1998); Sroufe et al., *The Development of the Person*.

51. Vaillant, *The Natural History of Alcoholism Revisited*, 171.

52. Ibid., 177–78.

53. Ibid., 172–73.

54. All the findings reported have statistical significance of < 0.05, i.e., less than a 5 percent probability of occurring by chance alone.

55. Vaillant, *The Natural History of Alcoholism Revisited*, table 3.9, 173.

56. Ibid., 179–81.

57. Lee Robins, *Deviant Children Grown Up* (Baltimore: The Williams and Wilkins Company, 1966), 73.

THREE. THE STING OF STIGMA

1. Betty Ford, "Testimony before Join Together Policy Panel," in *Ending Discrimination against People with Alcohol and Drug Problems: Recommendations from a National Policy Panel*, ed. Join Together (Boston: Boston University School of Public Health, 2002).

2. Gerhard Falk, *Stigma: How We Treat Outsiders* (Amherst, NY: Prometheus Books, 2001).

3. Ibid., 181.

4. Robin Room, "Stigma, Social Inequality and Alcohol and Drug Use," *Drug and Alcohol Review* 24, no. 2 (2005).

5. Michael Lemanski, *A History of Addiction and Recovery in the United States* (Tucson, AZ: See Sharp Press, 2001), 22.

6. John J. Rumbarger, *Profits, Power, and Prohibition: Alcohol Reform and the Indus-

trializing of America, 1800–1930, SUNY Series in New Social Studies on Alcohol and Drugs (Albany: State University of New York Press, 1989), 109; W. J. Rorabaugh, *The Alcoholic Republic: An American Tradition* (New York: Oxford University Press, 1979), 205.

7. Andrew Barr, *Drink: A Social History of America* (New York: Carroll & Graf Publishers, 2000), 1–14.

8. Genevieve M. Ames, "American Beliefs about Alcoholism: Historical Perspectives on the Medical-Moral Controversy," in *The American Experience with Alcohol*, ed. Linda A. Bennett and Genevieve M. Ames (New York: Plenum, 1985), 23–39.

9. Rorabaugh, *The Alcoholic Republic*, 8, 9, 28.

10. David F. Musto, *The American Disease: Origins of Narcotic Control*, 3rd ed. (New York: Oxford University Press, 1999), 5–8.

11. Ibid., 3.

12. Coca Cola Company, accessed Jun 5, 2013, www.coca-colacompany.com.

13. Jason Hughes, *Learning to Smoke: Tobacco Use in the West* (Chicago: University of Chicago Press, 2003), 94; Jordan Goodman, *Tobacco in History: The Cultures of Dependence*, paperback ed. (London: Routledge, 1994), 117.

14. *Harrison Narcotics Tax Act*, Public Law 223, 63rd Congress (Dec 14, 1914).

15. *U.S. v. Doremus*, 86 U.S. 249 (1919).

16. *Webb v. U.S.*, 249 U.S. 96 (1919).

17. Buprenorphine is a medication to prevent withdrawal and blunt craving in opiate-addicted patients. Since 2002, any physician completing eight hours of special training can apply for a federal waiver from the Harrison Act and treat opiate addiction in her office.

18. Teresa E. Seeman et al., "Social Network Ties and Mortality among the Elderly in the Alameda County Study," *American Journal of Epidemiology* 126, no. 4 (1987); Joe Tomaka, Sharon Thompson, and Rebecca Palacios, "The Relation of Social Isolation, Loneliness, and Social Support to Disease Outcomes among the Elderly," *Journal of Aging and Health* 18, no. 3 (2006).

19. K. R. Collins, "EAP Cost/Benefit Analyses: The Last Word," *EAPA Exchange* (Nov–Dec 2000).

20. Susan Rook, Join Together witness, in Join Together Policy Panel, Kurt L. Schmoke Esq., chair, "Ending Discrimination against People with Alcohol and Drug Problems" (Boston University School of Public Health, 2003).

21. Richard A. Rettig and Adam Yarmolinsky, eds., *Federal Regulation of Methadone Treatment, Institute of Medicine* (Washington, DC: National Academies Press, 1995), 29.

22. Daniel Chandler, *The Act of Writing: A Media Theory Approach* (Dyfed, Wales, UK: The Registry, 1995).

23. Author's personal experience, 1977–81.

24. Benjamin Rush, *An Inquiry into the Effects of Ardent Spirits upon the Human Body and Mind*, 6th ed. (New York: Lorig, 1811).

25. R. Finn and J. Clancy, "Alcoholism, Dilemma or Disease: A Recurring Problem for the Physician," *Comprehensive Psychiatry* 13, no. 2 (1972); J. N. Chappel and S. H. Schnoll, "Physician Attitudes: Effect on the Treatment of Chemically Dependent Patients," *JAMA* 237, no. 21 (1977).

26. Joseph C. Fisher et al., "Physicians and Alcoholics: The Effect of Medical Training on Attitudes Toward Alcoholics," *Journal of Studies on Alcohol and Drugs* 36, no. 7 (1975).

27. M. E. Rohman et al., "The Response of Primary Care Physicians to Problem Drinkers," *American Journal of Drug and Alcohol Abuse* 13, no. 1–2 (1987).

28. K. A. Bradley et al., "Primary and Secondary Prevention of Alcohol Problems: U.S. Internist Attitudes and Practices," *Journal of General Internal Medicine* 10, no. 2 (1995).

29. G. B. Wilson et al., "Intervention against Excessive Alcohol Consumption in Primary Health Care: A Survey of GPs' Attitudes and Practices in England 10 Years On," *Alcohol and Alcoholism* 46, no. 5 (2011).

30. Natalie Skinner et al., "Stigma and Discrimination in Health-Care Provision to Drug Users: The Role of Values, Affect, and Deservingness Judgments," *Journal of Applied Social Psychology* 37, no. 1 (2007).

31. Lars Hansson et al., "Mental Health Professionals' Attitudes Towards People with Mental Illness: Do They Differ from Attitudes Held by People with Mental Illness?" *International Journal of Social Psychiatry* 59, no. 1 (2013).

32. J. O. Merrill et al., "Mutual Mistrust in the Medical Care of Drug Users: The Keys to the "Narc" Cabinet," *Journal of General Internal Medicine* 17, no. 5 (2002).

33. Personal communication, David Rosenbloom, 2007.

34. Join Together Policy Panel, "Ending Discrimination."

35. Mary R. Haack and Adger Hoover, Jr., eds., "Strategic Plan for Interdisciplinary Faculty Development: Arming the Nation's Health Professional Workforce for a New Approach to Substance Use Disorders," *Substance Abuse* 23, no. 3, suppl (2002); Ernest Rasyidi, Jeffery N. Wilkins, and Itai Danovitch, "Training the Next Generation of Providers in Addiction Medicine," *Psychiatric Clinics of North America* 35, no. 2 (2012).

36. Hansson et al., "Mental Health Professionals' Attitudes"

37. Jennifer Friedman and Marixsa Alicea, *Surviving Heroin: Interviews with Women in Methadone Clinics* (Gainesville: University Press of Florida, 2001). 152–53, 55.

38. Ibid., 132–33, 137, 152–53.

39. Jacqueline Smith-Darling (1956–2004), with permission from her husband, Albert Darling.

40. Deborah S. Hasin et al., "Prevalence, Correlates, Disability, and Comorbidity of DSM-IV Alcohol Abuse and Dependence in the United States: Results from the National Epidemiologic Survey on Alcohol and Related Conditions," *Archives of General Psychiatry* 64, no. 7 (2007).

41. Norman Miller et al., "Why Physicians Are Unprepared."

42. Vaillant, *The Natural History of Alcoholism*, 190.

43. Brent Egan, Yumin Zhao, and Neal Axon, "U.S. Trends in Prevalence, Awareness, Treatment, and Control of Hypertension," *JAMA* 303, no. 20 (2010).

44. Centers for Disease Control and Prevention, "National Diabetes Fact Sheet: National Information on Diabetes and Prediabetes in the United States, 2011," ed. U.S. Department of Health and Human Services (Atlanta, 2011).

45. CASAColumbia, "Addiction Medicine: Closing the Gap between Science and Practice" (New York: The National Center on Addiction and Substance Abuse at Columbia University [CASAColumbiaTM], 2012).

46. A. M. Miniño and S. L. Murphy, "Death in the United States, 2010" (Hyattsville, MD, 2012).

47. American Heart Association, "Annual Report" (2009), accessed Feb 27, 2012, www.heart.org; National Institutes of Health, "The NIH Almanac," NIH, accessed Jun 2, 2013, www.nih.gov.

48. "The Addiction Recovery Guide," accessed Jun 2, 2013, www.addiction recoveryguide.org.

49. T. D'Aunno and H. A. Pollack, "Changes in Methadone Treatment Practices: Results from a National Panel Study, 1988–2000," *JAMA* 288, no. 7 (2002).

50. Norman Miller et al., "Why Physicians Are Unprepared."

51. Haack and Hoover, eds., "Strategic Plan."

52. U.S. Institute of Medicine, *Broadening the Base of Treatment for Alcohol Problems* (Washington, DC: National Academies Press, 1990).

53. Marianne T. Marcus, "Final Progress Report. HRSA-AMERSA-SAMHSA/CSAT Interdisciplinary Program to Improve Health Professional Education in Substance Abuse. Grant No.: 1U78 HP 00001–03," (Providence, RI: Association for Medical Education and Research in Substance Abuse [AMERSA], 2006).

54. CASAColumbia, "Addiction Medicine."

55. Roland Sturm, Weiying Zhang, and Michael Schoenbaum, "How Expensive Are Unlimited Substance Abuse Benefits under Managed Care?" *Journal of Behavioral Health Services & Research* 26, no. 2 (1999).

56. U.S. Department of Labor, "Fact Sheet: The Mental Health Parity and Addiction Equity Act of 2008 (MHPAEA)," U.S. Department of Labor, accessed Jun 5, 2013, www.dol.gov/.

57. *Patient Protection and Affordable Care Act of 2010*, Public Law no. 111–148, 124 Stat. 119 (2010).

58. Victor A. Capoccia et al., "Massachusetts's Experience Suggests Coverage Alone Is Insufficient to Increase Addiction Disorders Treatment," *Health Affairs (Millwood)* 31, no. 5 (2012).

59. American Society of Addiction Medicine, "Advancing Access to Addiction Medications: Implications for Opioid Addiction Treatment," (2013), accessed Mar 28, 2014, www.asam.org/docs/advocacy/Implications-for-Opioid-Addiction-Treatment.

60. Ellen M. Weber, " Equality Standards for Health Insurance Coverage: Will the Mental Health Parity and Addiction Equity Act End the Discrimination" (2012), *Golden Gate University Law Review* 43, no. 2 (2013); American Society of Addiction Medicine, "Advancing Access."

61. Personal communication with Deb Beck, Jun 01, 2007.

62. David U. Himmelstein et al., "Medical Bankruptcy in the United States, 2007: Results of a National Study," *American Journal of Medicine* 122, no. 8 (2009).

63. Christine R. Stehman and Mark B. Mycyk, "A Rational Approach to the Treatment of Alcohol Withdrawal in the ED," *American Journal of Emergency Medicine* 31, no. 4 (2013); E. Jennifer Edelman et al., "Combining Rapid HIV Testing and a Brief Alcohol Intervention in Young Unhealthy Drinkers in the Emergency Department: A Pilot Study," *American Journal of Drug and Alcohol Abuse* 38, no. 6 (2012); Gail D'Onofrio et al., "A Brief Intervention Reduces Hazardous and Harmful Drinking in Emergency Department Patients," *Annals of Emergency Medicine* 60, no. 2 (2012).

64. *Contract with America Advancement Act of 1996,* Public Law. no 104-121, 110 Stat. 847 (1996).

65. *Personal Responsibility and Work Opportunity Reconciliation Act,* Public Law no. 104-193, Sect. 115, 110 Stat. 2105 (1996).

66. Federal Student Aid, an office of the U.S. Department of Education, "Incarcerated Individuals and Eligibility for Federal Student Aid," ed. Federal Student Aid, accessed Jun 5, 2013, http://studentaid.ed.gov/sites/default/files/aid-info-for-incarcerated-individuals.pdf.

67. U.S. Department of Health and Human Services, "Healthy People 2020: Topics and Objectives," U.S. Department of Health and Human Services, accessed Jun 5, 2013, www.healthypeople.gov.

68. Join Together Policy Panel, "Ending Discrimination"; Roberta Leis and David Rosenbloom, "The Road from Addiction Recovery to Productivity: Ending Discrimination against People with Alcohol and Drug Problems," *Family Court Review* 47 (2009).

69. Center for Public Advocacy, "National Study of Public Attitudes toward Addiction, 2008," (Center City, MN: Hazelden, 2008).

FOUR. RISK AND RESILIENCE

1. Michael Rutter, "Implications of Resilience Concepts for Scientific Understanding," *Annals of the New York Academy of Sciences* 1094 (2006).

2. Sroufe et al., *The Development of the Person.*

3. William Shakespeare, *The Tragedy of Hamlet,* The Kittredge Shakespeare, ed. George L. Kittredge (Boston: Ginn, 1939).

4. M. T. Bardo et al., "Environmental Enrichment Decreases Intravenous Self-Administration of Amphetamine in Female and Male Rats," *Psychopharmacology (Berl)* 155, no. 3 (2001); Erwan Bezard et al., "Enriched Environment Confers Resistance to 1-Methyl-4-Phenyl-1,2,3,6-Tetrahydropyridine and Cocaine: Involvement of Dopamine Transporter and Trophic Factors," *Journal of Neuroscience* 23, no. 35 (2003).

5. C. D. Drews et al., "The Relationship between Idiopathic Mental Retardation and Maternal Smoking during Pregnancy," *Pediatrics* 97, no. 4 (1996).

6. G. Koren et al., "Fetal Alcohol Spectrum Disorder," *CMAJ* 169, no. 11 (2003).

7. P. S. Cook et al., "Alcohol, Tobacco and Other Drugs May Harm the Unborn," ed. U.S. Department of Health and Human Services, Pub. No. (ADM) 90-1711 (U.S. Department of Health and Human Services [USDHHS], 1990).

8. J. L. Johnson and M. Leff, "Children of Substance Abusers: Overview of Research Findings," *Pediatrics* 1035, no. part 2 (1999).

9. Sroufe et al., *The Development of the Person.*

10. Michael J. Meaney, "Maternal Care, Gene Expression, and the Transmission of Individual Differences in Stress Reactivity across Generations," *Annual Review of Neuroscience* 24 (2001).

11. Arnold J. Sameroff and Katherine L. Rosenblum, "Psychosocial Constraints on the Development of Resilience," *Annals of the New York Academy of Sciences* 1094 (2006).

12. Karen Appleyard et al., "When More Is Not Better: The Role of Cumulative Risk in Child Behavior Outcomes," *Journal of Child Psychology and Psychiatry* 46, no. 3 (2005).

13. Stuart T. Hauser, Joseph P. Allen, and Eve Golden, *Out of the Woods: Tales of Resilient Teens* (Cambridge: Harvard University Press, 2006), 285.

14. David A. Kessler, *A Question of Intent: A Great American Battle with a Deadly Industry* (Cambridge, MA: The Perseus Books Group, 2001), 275–79.

15. Mary-Anne Enoch, "Genetic and Environmental Influences on the Development of Alcoholism: Resilience vs. Risk," *Annals of the New York Academy of Sciences* 1094 (2006).

16. Linda Spear, "The Teenage Brain: Adolescents and Alcohol," *Current Directions in Psychological Science* 22, no. 2 (2013).

17. William Wordsworth, "My Heart Leaps Up (1807)," in *The Norton Anthology of English Literature*, ed. M. H. Abrams (New York: W. W. Norton & Company, 1962).

18. Y. L. Hurd, "Perspectives on Current Directions in the Neurobiology of Addiction Disorders Relevant to Genetic Risk Factors," *CNS Spectrums* 11, no. 11 (2006).

19. David Kalman, Sandra Baker Morissette, and Tony P. George, "Co-morbidity of Smoking in Patients with Psychiatric and Substance Use Disorders," *American Journal on Addictions* 14, no. 2 (2005).

20. Thomas J. Crowley and Paula D. Riggs, "Adolescent Substance Use Disorder with Conduct Disorder and Comorbid Conditions," in *National Institute on Drug Abuse Research Monograph No. 156,* ed. Elizabeth Rahdert and Dorynne Czechowicz (Rockville, MD: National Institutes of Health, Public Health Service, U.S. Department of Health and Human Services, 1995); William G. Iacono, Stephen M. Malone, and Matt McGue, "Behavioral Disinhibition and the Development of Early-Onset Addiction: Common and Specific Influences," *Annual Review of Clinical Psychology* 4 (2008).

21. Marsha E. Bates and Erich W. Labouvie, "Adolescent Risk Factors and the Prediction of Persistent Alcohol and Drug Use into Adulthood," *Alcoholism: Clinical and Experimental Research* 21, no. 5 (1997).

22. Kathleen T. Brady and Rajita Sinha, "Co-occurring Mental and Substance Use Disorders: The Neurobiological Effects of Chronic Stress," *American Journal of Psychiatry* 162, no. 8 (2005).

23. Bates and Labouvie, "Adolescent Risk Factors."

24. Jane Stewart, "Stress and Relapse to Drug Seeking: Studies in Laboratory Animals Shed Light on Mechanisms and Sources of Long-Term Vulnerability," *American Journal on Addictions* 12, no. 1 (2003).

25. Ibid.

26. Ming D. Li and Margit Burmeister, "New Insights into the Genetics of Addiction," *Nature Reviews Genetics* 10 (2009).

27. Avshalom Caspi et al., "Role of Genotype in the Cycle of Violence in Maltreated Children," *Science* 297 (2002).

28. Andrew J. Saxon, Michael R. Oreskovich, and Zoran Brkanac, "Genetic Determinants of Addiction to Opioids and Cocaine," *Harvard Review of Psychiatry* 13, no. 4 (2005).

29. Avshalom Caspi et al., "Moderation of the Effect of Adolescent-Onset Cannabis Use on Adult Psychosis by a Functional Polymorphism in the Catechol-O-Methyltransferase Gene: Longitudinal Evidence of a Gene X Environment Interaction," *Biological Psychiatry* 57, no. 10 (2005).

30. Mary Jeanne Kreek et al., "Genetic Influences on Impulsivity, Risk Taking,

Stress Responsivity and Vulnerability to Drug Abuse and Addiction," *Nature Neuroscience* 8, no. 11 (2005).

31. Brady and Sinha, "Co-occurring Mental and Substance Use Disorders."

32. Nora D. Volkow et al., "Addiction Circuitry in the Human Brain," *Annual Review of Pharmacology and Toxicology* 52 (2012).

33. Michael Rutter, *Genes and Behavior: Nature-Nurture Interplay Explained* (Oxford, UK: Blackwell Publishing, 2006); Brady and Sinha, "Co-occurring Mental and Substance Use Disorders."

34. Rutter, 175–182.

35. Michael Rutter, "Developmental Catch-up, and Deficit, Following Adoption after Severe Global Early Privation," *Journal of Child Psychology and Psychiatry* 39, no. 4 (1998).

36. Ann S. Masten and Anne Shaffer, "How Families Matter in Child Development: Reflections from Research on Risk and Resilience," in *Families Count: Effects of Child and Adolescent Development*, ed. Alison Clarke-Stewart and Judy Dunn (New York: Cambridge University Press, 2006).

37. Sameroff and Rosenblum, "Psychosocial Constraints."

38. Michael Rutter, "The Promotion of Resilience in the Face of Adversity," in *Families Count: Effects on Child and Adolescent Development,* ed. Alison Clarke-Stewart and Judy Dunn (New York: Cambridge University Press, 2006).

39. Kenneth J. Sher et al., "The Role of Childhood Stressors in the Intergenerational Transmission of Alcohol Use Disorders," *Journal of Studies on Alcohol and Drugs* 58, no. 4 (1997).

40. Joe Westermeyer et al., "Substance Use Disorder among Adoptees: A Clinical Comparative Study," *American Journal of Drug and Alcohol Abuse* 33, no. 3 (2007).

41. C. R. Cloninger, M. Bohman, and S. Sigvardsson, "Inheritance of Alcohol Abuse: Cross-Fostering Analysis of Adopted Men," *Archives of General Psychiatry* 38 (1981).

42. Sroufe et al., *The Development of the Person.*

43. John R. Knight et al., "A New Brief Screen for Adolescent Substance Abuse," *Archives of Pediatrics & Adolescent Medicine* 153, no. 6 (1999).

44. John R. Knight et al., "Prevalence of Positive Substance Abuse Screen Results among Adolescent Primary Care Patients," *Archives of Pediatrics and Adolescent Medicine* 161, no. 11 (2007).

45. Englund, unpublished data 2006.

46. Malcolm Gladwell, *The Tipping Point: How Little Things Can Make a Big Difference* (Boston: Back Bay Books, 2002).

47. Bob Dylan, *Lyrics, 1962–2001* (New York: Simon & Schuster, 2004).

48. Hauser, Allen, and Golden, *Out of the Woods.*

FIVE. RECOVERY: OWNING THE TREATMENT AND THE OUTCOMES

The epigraph to chapter 5 is from Kate R. Lorig and Halsted R. Holman, "Self-Management Education: History, Definition, Outcomes, and Mechanisms," *Annals of Behavioral Medicine* 26, no. 1 (2003); see also Richard Saitz et al., "The Case for Chronic Disease Management for Addiction," *Journal of Addiction Medicine* 2, no. 2 (2008).

1. U.S. Institute of Medicine, Committee on Crossing the Quality Chasm: Ad-

aptation to Mental Health and Addictive Disorders, *Improving the Quality of Health Care for Mental and Substance-Use Conditions,* Quality Chasm Series, ed. Institute of Medicine (Washington, DC: The National Academies Press, 2006), 38.

2. Miniño and Murphy. "Death in the United States."

3. Lorig and Holman, "Self-Management Education."

4. Henry R. Kranzler and Richard N. Rosenthal, "Dual Diagnosis: Alcoholism and Co-morbid Psychiatric Disorders," *American Journal on Addictions* 12 suppl 1 (2003); *U.S. v. Doremus.*

5. Kessler, *A Question of Intent;* David A. Kessler et al., "Nicotine Addiction: A Pediatric Disease," *Journal of Pediatrics* 130, no. 4 (1997).

6. Alex Wodak and Annie Cooney, "Do Needle Syringe Programs Reduce HIV Infection among Injecting Drug Users: A Comprehensive Review of the International Evidence," *Substance Use & Misuse* 41, no. 6–7 (2006); P. Anderson, D. Chisholm, and D. C. Fuhr, "Effectiveness and Cost-Effectiveness of Policies and Programmes to Reduce the Harm Caused by Alcohol," *Lancet* 373, no. 9682 (2009).

7. D. E. Logan and G. A. Marlatt, "Harm Reduction Therapy: A Practice-Friendly Review of Research," *Journal of Clinical Psychology* 66, no. 2 (2010); Wodak and Cooney, "Do Needle Syringe Programs Reduce HIV Infection; Anderson, Chisholm, and Fuhr, "Effectiveness and Cost-Effectiveness."

8. G. A. Marlatt, "Taxonomy of High Risk Situations for Alcohol Relapse: Evolution of a Cognitive-Behavioral Model," *Addiction* 91 suppl (1996).

9. Ronald C. Kessler, "The Epidemiology of Dual Diagnosis," *Biological Psychiatry* 56, no. 10 (2004).

10. Linda B. Cottler et al., "Posttraumatic Stress Disorder among Substance Users from the General Population," *American Journal of Psychiatry* 149, no. 5 (1992); Louise Langman and Man Cheung Chung, "The Relationship between Forgiveness, Spirituality, Traumatic Guilt and Posttraumatic Stress Disorder (PTSD) among People with Addiction," *Psychiatric Quarterly* (2013).

11. Geoffrey Williams et al., "Reducing the Health risks of Diabetes: How self-determination Theory May Help Improve Medication Theory and Quality of Life," *Diabetes Educator* 35, no. 3 (2009).

12. Paulo Freire, "Impossible to Exist without Dreams," in *Daring to Dream: Toward a Pedagogy of the Unfinished,* ed. Donald Macedo (Boulder, CO: Paradigm Publishers, 2004).

13. Lorig and Holman, "Self-management Education"; Theresa W. Kim et al., "Effect of Quality Chronic Disease Management for Alcohol and Drug Dependence on Addiction Outcomes," *Journal of Substance Abuse Treatment* 43, no. 4 (2012).

14. William R. Miller and Stephen Rollnick, *Motivational Interviewing: Preparing People for Change,* 2nd ed. (New York: Guilford Press, 2002).

15. Paulo Freire, *Pedagogy of the Oppressed,* trans. Myra Bergman Ramos (New York: Seabury Press, 1970 [1968]).

16. James O. Prochaska and Carlo C. DiClemente, "Stages and Process of Self Change in Smoking: Toward an Integrative Model of Change," *Journal of Consulting and Clinical Psychology* 51 (1983).

17. Jeffrey H. Samet and Patrick G. O'Connor, "Alcohol Abusers in Primary Care: Readiness to Change Behavior," *American Journal of Medicine* 105, no. 4 (1998).

18. Lee Ann Kaskutas, "Alcoholics Anonymous Effectiveness: Faith Meets Science," *Journal of Addictive Diseases* 28, no. 2 (2009).

19. Rudolf H. Moos and Bernice S. Moos, "Participation in Treatment and Alcoholics Anonymous: A 16-Year Follow-up of Initially Untreated Individuals," *Journal of Clinical Psychology* 62, no. 6 (2006).

20. Jon Morgenstern et al, "Examining Mechanisms of Action in 12-Step Treatment: The Role of 12-Step Cognitions," *Journal of Studies on Alcohol* 63, no. 6 (2002): 665–72.

21. Jon F. Kelly et. al., "How Do People Recover from Alcohol Dependence? A Systematic Review of the Research on Mechanisms of Behavioral Change in Alcoholics Anonymous," *Addiction Research and Theory* 17, no. 3 (2009): 236–59.

22. Morgenstern et. al., "Examining Mechanisms of Action."

23. William Carlos Williams, *The Autobiography of William Carlos Williams* (New York: New Directions Books, 1951); Samet and O'Connor, "Alcohol Abusers," 361–62.

24. U.S. Institute of Medicine, Committee on Crossing the Quality Chasm, *Improving the Quality of Health Care*, chap. 1, 29–55.

25. Constance Weisner et al., "Short-Term Alcohol and Drug Treatment Outcomes Predict Long-Term Outcome," *Drug and Alcohol Dependence* 71, no. 3 (2003); Janice Y. Tsoh et al., "Stopping Smoking during First Year of Substance Use Treatment Predicted 9-Year Alcohol and Drug Treatment Outcomes," *Drug and Alcohol Dependence* 114, no. 2 (2011).

26. William R. Miller, Scott T. Walters, and Melanie E. Bennett, "How Effective Is Alcoholism Treatment in the United States?" *Journal of Studies on Alcohol and Drugs* 62, no. 2 (2001).

27. Michael L. Prendergast et al., "The Effectiveness of Drug Abuse Treatment: A Meta-analysis of Comparison Group Studies," *Drug and Alcohol Dependence* 67 (2002).

28. William R. Miller, R. Gayle Benefield, and J. Scott Tonigan, "Enhancing Motivation for Change in Problem Drinking: A Controlled Comparison of Two Therapist Styles," *Journal of Consulting and Clinical Psychology* 61 (1993).

29. Constance Weisner et al., "Who Goes to Alcohol and Drug Treatment? Understanding Utilization within the Context of Insurance," *Journal of Studies on Alcohol and Drugs* 63 (2002); T. Cameron Wild, Jody Wolfe, and Elaine Hyshka, "Consent and Coercion in Addiction Treatment," *Addiction Neuroethics: The Ethics of Addiction Neuroscience Research and Treatment* (2012).

30. T. Cameron Wild, Amanda B. Roberts, and Erin L. Cooper, "Compulsory Substance Abuse Treatment: An Overview of Recent Findings and Issues," *European Addiction Research* 8, no. 2 (2002).

31. Jennifer L. Skeem, John Encandela, and Jennifer Eno Louden, "Perspectives on Probation and Mandated Mental Health Treatment in Specialized and Traditional Probation Departments," *Behavioral Sciences and the Law* 21 (2003).

32. A. Thomas McLellan and Kathleen Meyers, "Contemporary Addiction Treatment: A Review of Systems Problems for Adults and Adolescents," *Biological Psychiatry* 56, no. 10 (2004).

33. U.S. Institute of Medicine, Committee on Crossing the Quality Chasm, *Improving the Quality of Health Care*.

34. Elizabeth A. McGlynn et al., "The Quality of Health Care Delivered to Adults in the United States," *New England Journal of Medicine* 348, no. 26 (2003); CASA Columbia, "Addiction Medicine."

35. U.S. Institute of Medicine, *Broadening the Base*, 212.

36. WHO Brief Intervention Study Group, "A Randomized Cross-National Clinical Trial of Brief Intervention with Heavy Drinkers," *American Journal Public Health* 86, no. 7 (1996).

37. Leif I. Solberg, Michael V. Maciosek, and Nichol M. Edwards, "Primary Care Intervention to Reduce Alcohol Misuse: Ranking Its Health Impact and Cost Effectiveness," *American Journal of Preventive Medicine* 34, no. 2 (2008); Michael F. Fleming et al., "Benefit-Cost Analysis of Brief Physician Advice with Problem Drinkers in Primary Care Settings," *Medical Care* 38, no. 1 (2000).

38. Nicolas Bertholet et al., "Reduction of Alcohol Consumption by Brief Alcohol Intervention in Primary Care: Systematic Review and Meta-analysis," *Archives of Internal Medicine* 165, no. 9 (2005).

39. Lorig and Holman, "Self-management Education."

40. Judith Bernstein et al., "Brief Motivational Intervention at a Clinic Visit Reduces Cocaine and Heroin Use," *Drug and Alcohol Dependence* 77 (2005); Richard S. Garfein et al., "A Peer-Education Intervention to Reduce Injection Risk Behaviors for HIV and Hepatitis C Virus Infection in Young Injection Drug Users," *Aids* 21, no. 14 (2007).

41. U.S. Institute of Medicine, Committee on Crossing the Quality Chasm, *Improving the Quality of Health Cares*.

42. Haack and Adger, eds., "Strategic Plan."

43. Franklin Delano Roosevelt, "Second Inaugural Address" (Washington, DC, 1937).

SIX. DRUGS FOR DRUGS

1. Centers for Disease Control and Prevention, National Center for Injury Prevention and Control, Division of Unintentional Injury Prevention, "Drug Overdose in the United States: Fact Sheet, accessed Jan 8, 2014, www.cdc.gov/homeandre creationalsafety/overdose/fact.html; Centers for Disease Control and Prevention, "Vital Signs: Overdoses of Prescription Opioid Pain Relievers—United States, 1998–2008," *Morbidity and Mortality Weekly Report* 60 no. 43 (2011), accessed May 12, 2013, www.cdc.gov.; Centers for Disease Control and Prevention, "Motor Vehicle-Related Death Rates—United States, 1999–2005," *Morbidity and Mortality Weekly Report* 58 (2009).

2. "Community-Based Opioid Overdose Prevention Programs Providing Naloxone—United States, 2010," *Morbidity Mortality Weekly Report* 61, no. 6 (2012).

3. Jackie MacMullan, *Boston Globe* (Jun 25, 1986).

4. American Psychiatric Association, *Diagnostic and Statistical Manual of Mental Disorders* (DSM-IV-TR).

5. Mary Jeanne Kreek, personal communication, Dec 2006.

6. Henrietta N. Barnes, Mark D. Aronson, and Thomas L. Delbanco, *Alcoholism: A Guide for the Primary Care Physician*, ed. Mack Lipkin, Frontiers of Primary Care (New York: Springer-Verlag, 1987).

7. J. C. Hughes and C. C. Cook, "The Efficacy of Disulfiram: A Review of Outcome Studies," *Addiction* 92, no. 4 (1997).

8. Vincent P. Dole, "Narcotic Addiction, Physical Dependence and Relapse," *New England Journal of Medicine* 286, no. 18 (1972).

9. Susan M. Stine and Thomas R. Kosten, "Pharmacologic Interventions for Opioid Dependence," in *Principles of Addiction Medicine, Fourth Edition*, ed. Richard K. Ries et al. (Philadelphia: Lippincott, Williams, & Wilkins, 2009), 659.

10. Tove S. Rosen and Helen L. Johnson, "Long-Term Effects of Prenatal Methadone Maintenance," National Institute on Drug Abuse (NIDA) Monograph 59 (1985).

11. Barry Stimmel et al., "Ability to Remain Abstinent after Methadone Detoxification.: A Six-Year Study," *JAMA* 237, no. 12 (1977).

12. Paul Cushman, Jr., "Abstinence Following Detoxification and Methadone Maintenance Treatment," *American Journal of Medicine* 65, no. 1 (1978).

13. U.S. Food and Drug Administration, "Nicotine Replacement Therapy Labels May Change," Department of Health and Human Services, accessed Jul 21, 2013, www.fda.gov.

14. John A. Dani, Thomas R. Kosten, and Neal L. Benowitz, "The Pharmacology of Nicotine and Tobacco," in *Principles of Addiction Medicine*, ed. Richard K. Ries, D. A. Fiellin, and Shannon C. Miller (Philadelphia: Lippincott, Williams & Wilkins, 2009), 183.

15. Karen Lasser et al., "Smoking and Mental Illness: A Population-Based Prevalence Study," *JAMA* 284, no. 20 (2000).

16. Manit Srisurapanont and Ngamwong Jarusuraisin, "Naltrexone for the Treatment of Alcoholism: A Meta-analysis of Randomized Controlled Trials," *International Journal of Neuropsychopharmacology* 8, no. 2 (2005).

17. Henry R. Kranzler and Allyson Gage, "Acamprosate Efficacy in Alcohol-Dependent Patients: Summary of Results from Three Pivotal Trials," *American Journal on Addictions* 17, no. 1 (2008).

18. Falk Kiefer et al., "Comparing and Combining Naltrexone and Acamprosate in Relapse Prevention of Alcoholism: A Double-Blind, Placebo-Controlled Study," *Archives of General Psychiatry* 60, no. 1 (2003).

19. Kristin V. Carson et al., "Current and Emerging Pharmacotherapeutic Options for Smoking Cessation," *Substance Abuse: Research and Treatment* 7 (2013).

20. N. A. Rigotti, "Strategies to Help a Smoker Who Is Struggling to Quit," *JAMA* 308, no. 15 (2012).

21. Henry R. Kranzler, Domenic A. Ciraulo, and Jerome H. Jaffe, "Medications for Use in Alcohol Rehabilitation," in *Principles of Addiction Medicine*, ed. Richard K. Ries et al. (Philadelphia: Lippincott, Williams & Wilkins, 2009).

22. B. A. Johnson et al., "Topiramate for Treating Alcohol Dependence: A Randomized Controlled Trial," *JAMA* 298, no. 14 (2007).

EPILOGUE

1. Michael Balint, "The Doctor, his Patient, and the Illness," *Lancet* 265, no. 6866 (1955).

GLOSSARY

alcohol use disorder (AUD). A pattern of persistent alcohol use despite negative consequences. AUD may be described as "mild," "moderate," or "severe," depending on the number of symptoms due to alcohol use and the number and severity of adverse outcomes (social, physical, mental, occupational).

Alcoholics Anonymous (AA). A worldwide fellowship of independent groups of people with AUD sharing their experiences of addiction and recovery in order to solve their alcohol problems and to help others with AUD recover. A desire to stop drinking is the only criterion for membership.

allele. Any one of several variations of a gene that occupies a specific locus on a chromosome.

alprazolam. A short-acting benzodiazepine with rapid onset of action (Xanax).

amygdala. A part of the brain's limbic system that processes emotions (fear, pleasure, anger) and related memories.

anterior cingulate cortex. A component of the brain's limbic system that modulates emotional behaviors (visceral reactions to fear or anger) through its effect on the autonomic and hormonal systems.

benzodiazepines. A class of addictive central nervous system depressants used to treat anxiety and sleep problems. These drugs are active at many of the same brain receptors as alcohol.

buprenorphine. A partial opioid agonist that suppresses withdrawal symptoms and craving in opioid-addicted people, without the same negative effects of respiratory depression and death associated with excessive use of full opioid agonists (oxycodone, morphine, methadone). Licensed by the U.S. Food and Drug Administration in 2002 to treat opioid addiction in physicians' offices.

cannabinoids. A class of diverse chemical compounds that activate cannabinoid receptors in the brain and affect the function of other neurotransmitters. This class includes chemicals normally produced by the human body (anandamide) and the plant cannabis (marijuana).

clonazepam. A benzodiazepine used for the treatment of anxiety disorders, frequently abused because of its rapid onset of action (Klonopin).

contiguity. In conditioning, the temporal relationship between a stimulus and reward; for effective conditioning, this relationship should be a matter of seconds.

contingency. In conditioning, contingency refers to the likelihood that a unique conditioned stimulus (seeing one's drug dealer) will be much more likely to

lead to a reward and, conversely, the reward is unlikely to occur unless preceded by the unique stimulus.

corticotropin releasing factor (CRF). A brain hormone, released by the hypothalamus and amygdala, responsible for initiating many of the hormonal,
autonomic, and behavioral reactions to stress. (See **hypothalamic-pituitary-
adrenal axis.**)

diazepam. A long-acting benzodiazepine used in treatment of alcohol withdrawal
and anxiety (Valium).

dopamine. The major neurotransmitter in the brain's limbic reward system, involved with learning and memory.

dorsal striatum. Area of the brain involved in the selection and initiation of automatic or habitual behaviors.

functional magnetic resonance imaging (fMRI). A brain-imaging procedure that
measures brain activity by detecting differences in blood flow to regions of the
brain.

hippocampus. A structure in the limbic system adjacent to the amygdala
involved in emotional responses, consolidation of memories, and spatial
orientation.

hypothalamic pituitary adrenal axis (HPA). A neurohormonal network that
transmits signals from the hypothalamus via the pituitary to the adrenal gland
to increase the output of the stress hormone cortisol.

hypothalamus. The limbic structure primarily responsible for homeostasis,
involving control of autonomic and endocrine functions. The hypothalamus
governs the intake of food, water, and sleep-wake cycles.

incentive salience. The degree of importance (wanting and liking) of a reward
that leads to increased (or decreased) motivation to pursue the reward.

limbic system. The group of interconnected brain structures related to basic survival behaviors, which processes emotions, motivations, and memories.

mesolimbic pathway. This dopaminergic system collects and processes neural
stimuli and connects to higher brain functions in the cortex. It is involved in
learning, wanting, and motivation. Structures in this system include the ventral tegmental area, amygdala, hippocampus, and nucleus accumbens.

methadone. A long-acting synthetic opioid used for the treatment of chronic pain
and opiate addiction.

methadone maintenance treatment (MMT). A highly regulated system for
dispensing methadone and providing counseling services for opiate-addicted
people.

Narcotics Anonymous (NA). For people addicted to narcotic or other illicit drugs.
(See **Alcoholics Anonymous.**)

neurotransmitter. The class of brain chemicals that send signals from one
brain cell to another across a synapse. Neurotransmitters can be excitatory or
inhibitory.

nucleus accumbens (NAc). Receives inputs from other parts of the brain and
from addictive drugs. It is involved in anticipation, wanting, motivation, and
facilitating goal-oriented behaviors.

office-based opioid treatment. Treatment of opioid addiction in an outpatient
setting by a physician licensed by the U.S. Drug Enforcement Agency to pre-

scribe buprenorphine. (In contrast to the more structured and regulated methadone maintenance programs.)

opiate. A chemical product derived solely from opium; includes codeine, morphine, and heroin.

opioid. The class of addictive analgesic drugs including opiates, semisynthetic opiates (oxycodone), and synthetic compounds with morphine-like activity (methadone, fentanyl).

orbitofrontal cortex (OFC). The part of the prefrontal cortex involved in cognitive processing and decision making related to emotions and rewards. It has reciprocal connections with the limbic system.

plasticity. In neuroscience, the capacity of the brain to alter its structures (and function) in response to stimuli and experience.

prediction error hypothesis. The theory that the "reward" system is a system of expectation, learning, and memory. An increase in dopamine indicates an experience was better than expected; a decrease, worse than expected; no change in dopamine, just as expected without any new learning.

prefrontal cortex (PFC). The executive function center of the brain involved in priority setting, self-control, personality expression, and planning of complex cognitive behaviors.

sedative drugs. A class of addictive drugs that cause lethargy, sleepiness, respiratory depression, and in an overdose, death. The main subcategories include opioid analgesics, benzodiazepines, and barbiturates.

significance. In statistics, a finding is considered significant when the probability that it has occurred just by chance is very low, e.g., less than 5 percent.

stimulant drugs. The diverse class of addictive drugs that have an activating effect on the brain (caffeine, nicotine, amphetamines, cocaine).

substance use disorders. The spectrum of problems related to the use of addictive substances. (See **alcohol use disorder.**)

substantia nigra. A structure in the midbrain with multiple functions, including reward seeking, learned responses to stimuli, motor control, and sleep-wake cycles.

ventral tegmental area. The part of the brain where most addictive drugs act to increase the output of dopamine to the mesolimbic system.

BIBLIOGRAPHY

Acheson, S. K., E. L. Ross, and H. S. Swartzwelder. "Age-Independent and Dose-Response Effects of Ethanol on Spatial Memory in Rats." *Alcohol* 23, no. 3 (Apr 2001): 167–75.

"The Addiction Recovery Guide." Accessed Jun 2, 2013. www.addictionrecovery guide.org.

"Addiction Science: From Molecules to Managed Care." National Institute on Drug Abuse. Accessed May 12, 2013. www.drugabuse.gov.

American Heart Association. "Annual Report" (2009). Accessed Feb 27, 2012. www.heart.org.

American Psychiatric Association. *Diagnostic and Statistical Manual of Mental Disorders.* 4th ed., text rev (DSM-IV-TR). Washington, DC: American Psychiatric Association, 2000.

American Society of Addiction Medicine. "Advancing Access to Addiction Medications: Implications for Opioid Addiction Treatment" (2013). Accessed Mar 28, 2014. www.asam.org/docs/advocacy/Implications-for-Opioid-Addiction -Treatment.

Ames, Genevieve M. "American Beliefs about Alcoholism: Historical Perspectives on the Medical-Moral Controversy." In *The American Experience with Alcohol,* edited by Linda A. Bennett and Genevieve M. Ames, 23–39. New York: Plenum, 1985.

Anderson, P., D. Chisholm, and D. C. Fuhr. "Effectiveness and Cost-Effectiveness of Policies and Programmes to Reduce the Harm Caused by Alcohol." *Lancet* 373, no. 9682 (Jun 27, 2009): 2234–46.

Appleyard, Karen, Byron Egeland, Manfred H. M. Dulmen, and L. Alan Sroufe. "When More Is Not Better: The Role of Cumulative Risk in Child Behavior Outcomes." *Journal of Child Psychology and Psychiatry* 46, no. 3 (Mar 2005): 235–45.

"Average for U.S. 2001–2005—Years of Potential Life Lost Due to Excessive Alcohol Use." Centers for Disease Control and Prevention. Accessed May 12, 2013. apps.nccd.cdc.gov.

Bandura, Albert. *Self-Efficacy: The Exercise of Control.* New York: W. H. Freeman & Company, 1997.

Bardo, M. T., J. E. Klebaur, J. M. Valone, and C. Deaton. "Environmental Enrichment Decreases Intravenous Self-administration of Amphetamine in Female and Male Rats." *Psychopharmacology (Berl)* 155, no. 3 (May 2001): 278–84.

Barnes, Henrietta N., Mark D. Aronson, and Thomas L. Delbanco. *Alcoholism: A Guide for the Primary Care Physician*. Frontiers of Primary Care. Edited by Mack Lipkin. New York: Springer-Verlag, 1987.

Barr, Andrew. *Drink: A Social History of America*. New York: Carroll & Graf Publishers, 2000.

Barron, Susan, Aaron White, H. Scott Swartzwelder, Richard L. Bell, Zachary A. Rodd, Craig J. Slawecki, Cindy L. Ehlers, et al. "Adolescent Vulnerabilities to Chronic Alcohol or Nicotine Exposure: Findings from Rodent Models." *Alcoholism: Clinical and Experimental Research* 29, no. 9 (Sep 2005): 1720–25.

Bates, Marsha E., and Erich W. Labouvie. "Adolescent Risk Factors and the Prediction of Persistent Alcohol and Drug Use into Adulthood." *Alcoholism: Clinical and Experimental Research* 21, no. 5 (Aug 1997): 944–50.

Berke, J. D., and S. E. Hyman. "Addiction, Dopamine, and the Molecular Mechanisms of Memory." *Neuron* 25, no. 3 (Mar 2000): 515–32.

Bernstein, Judith, Edward Bernstein, Katherine Tassiopoulos, Timothy Heeren, Suzette Levenson, and Ralph Hingson. "Brief Motivational Intervention at a Clinic Visit Reduces Cocaine and Heroin Use." *Drug and Alcohol Dependence* 77 (2005): 49–59.

Berridge, Kent C. "From Prediction Error to Incentive Salience: Mesolimbic Computation of Reward Motivation." *European Journal of Neuroscience* 35, no. 7 (Apr 2012): 1124–43.

Bertholet, Nicolas, Jean-Bernard Daeppen, Vincent Wietlisbach, Michael Fleming, and Bernard Burnand. "Reduction of Alcohol Consumption by Brief Alcohol Intervention in Primary Care: Systematic Review and Meta-analysis." *Archives of Internal Medicine* 165, no. 9 (2005): 986.

Bezard, Erwan, Sandra Dovero, David Belin, Sophie Duconger, Vernice Jackson-Lewis, Serge Przedborski, Pier Vincenzo Piazza, Christian E Gross, and Mohamed Jaber. "Enriched Environment Confers Resistance to 1-Methyl-4-Phenyl-1,2,3,6-Tetrahydropyridine and Cocaine: Involvement of Dopamine Transporter and Trophic Factors." *Journal of Neuroscience* 23, no. 35 (Dec 3, 2003): 999–1007.

Booth, Martin. *Opium: A History*. London: Simon & Schuster, 1996.

Bradley, K. A., S. J. Curry, T. D. Koepsell, and E. B. Larson. "Primary and Secondary Prevention of Alcohol Problems: U.S. Internist Attitudes and Practices." *Journal of General Internal Medicine* 10, no. 2 (Feb 1995): 67–72.

Brady, Kathleen T., and Rajita Sinha. "Co-occurring Mental and Substance Use Disorders: The Neurobiological Effects of Chronic Stress." *American Journal of Psychiatry* 162, no. 8 (Aug 2005): 1483–93.

Cahalan, D., and R. Room. "Problem Drinking among American Men Aged 21–59." *American Journal of Public Health* 62, no. 11 (Nov 1972): 1473–82.

Capoccia, Victor A., Kyle L. Grazier, Christopher Toal, James H. Ford, and David H. Gustafson. "Massachusetts's Experience Suggests Coverage Alone Is Insufficient to Increase Addiction Disorders Treatment." *Health Affairs (Millwood)* 31, no. 5 (May 2012): 1000–1008.

Carson, Kristin V., Malcolm P. Brinn, Thomas A. Robertson, Rachada To-A-Nan, Adrian J. Esterman, Matthew Peters, and Brian J. Smith. "Current and Emerging Pharmacotherapeutic Options for Smoking Cessation." *Substance Abuse: Research and Treatment* 7 (2013): 85–105.

CASAColumbia. "Addiction Medicine: Closing the Gap between Science and Practice." New York: The National Center on Addiction and Substance Abuse at Columbia University (CASAColumbiaTM), Jun 2012.

Casey, B. J., and Rebecca M. Jones. "Neurobiology of the Adolescent Brain and Behavior: Implications for Substance Use Disorders." *Journal of the American Academy of Child & Adolescent Psychiatry* 49, no. 12 (Dec 2010): 1189–201.

Casey, B. J., Nim Tottenham, Conor Liston, and Sarah Durston. "Imaging the Developing Brain: What Have We Learned about Cognitive Development?" *Trends in Cognitive Sciences* 9, no. 3 (Mar 2005): 104–10.

Casikar, V., E. Mujica, M. Mongelli, J. Aliaga, N. Lopez, C. Smith, and F. Bartholomew. "Does Chewing Coca Leaves Influence Physiology at High Altitude?" *Indian Journal of Clinical Biochemistry* 25, no. 3 (Jul 2010): 311–14.

Caspi, Avshalom, J. McClay, T. E. Moffitt, J. Mill, and I. W. Craig. "Role of Genotype in the Cycle of Violence in Maltreated Children." *Science* 297 (2002): 851–54.

Caspi, Avshalom, Terrie E. Moffitt, Mary Cannon, Joseph McClay, Robin Murray, HonaLee Harrington, Alan Taylor, et al. "Moderation of the Effect of Adolescent-Onset Cannabis Use on Adult Psychosis by a Functional Polymorphism in the Catechol-O-Methyltransferase Gene: Longitudinal Evidence of a Gene × Environment Interaction." *Biological Psychiatry* 57, no. 10 (May 15, 2005): 1117–27.

Center for Public Advocacy. "National Study of Public Attitudes toward Addiction, 2008." Center City, MN: Hazelden, 2008.

Centers for Disease Control and Prevention. "Motor Vehicle–Related Death Rates—United States, 1999–2005." *Morbidity and Mortality Weekly Report* 58 (2009): 161–65.

———. "National Diabetes Fact Sheet: National Information on Diabetes and Prediabetes in the United States, 2011." Edited by U.S. Department of Health and Human Services. Atlanta, 2011.

———. "Vital Signs: Overdoses of Prescription Opioid Pain Relievers—United States, 1998–2008." *Morbidity and Mortality Weekly Report* 60 no. 43 (2011): 1487–92. Accessed May 12, 2013. www.cdc.gov.

Cha, Young May, Qiang Li, Wilkie A. Wilson, and H. Scott Swartzwelder. "Sedative and GABAergic Effects of Ethanol on Male and Female Rats." *Alcoholism: Clinical and Experimental Research* 30, no. 1 (Jan 2006): 113–18.

Chandler, Daniel. *The Act of Writing: A Media Theory Approach.* Dyfed, Wales, UK: The Registry, 1995.

Chappel, J. N., and S. H. Schnoll. "Physician Attitudes: Effect on the Treatment of Chemically Dependent Patients." *JAMA* 237, no. 21 (May 23, 1977): 2318–19.

Cloninger, C. R. , M. Bohman, and S. Sigvardsson. "Inheritance of Alcohol Abuse: Cross-Fostering Analysis of Adopted Men." *Archives of General Psychiatry* 38 (1981): 861–69.

Coca Cola Company. Accessed Jun 5, 2013. www.coca-colacompany.com.

"Cocaine: Abuse and Addiction." National Institute on Drug Abuse. Accessed May 25, 2013. www.drugabuse.gov.

Collins, K. R. "EAP Cost/Benefit Analyses: The Last Word." *EAPA Exchange* (Nov–Dec 2000): 30–31.

Collins, Michael A., Edward J. Neafsey, Kenneth J. Mukamal, Mary O. Gray, Dale A. Parks, Dipak K. Das, and Ronald J. Korthuis. "Alcohol in Moderation, Cardioprotection, and Neuroprotection: Epidemiological Considerations and Mechanistic Studies." *Alcoholism: Clinical and Experimental Research* 33, no. 2 (Feb 2009): 206–19.

"Community-Based Opioid Overdose Prevention Programs Providing Naloxone— United States, 2010." *Morbidity Mortality Weekly Report* 61, no. 6 (Feb 17, 2012): 101–5.

Contract with America Advancement Act of 1996. Public Law 104-121, 110 Stat. 847 (1996).

Cook, P. S., et. al. "Alcohol, Tobacco and Other Drugs May Harm the Unborn." Edited by U.S. Department of Health and Human Services. Pub. No. (ADM) 90-1711, 17. U.S. Department of Health and Human Services (USDHHS), 1990.

Cottler, Linda B., Wilson M. Compton, Douglas Mager, Edward L. Spitznagel, and Aleksandar Janca. "Posttraumatic Stress Disorder among Substance Users from the General Population." *American Journal of Psychiatry* 149, no. 5 (May 1992): 664–70.

Crews, Fulton T., Christopher J. Braun, Blair Hoplight, Robert C. Switzer, and Darin J. Knapp. "Binge Ethanol Consumption Causes Differential Brain Damage in Young Adolescent Rats Compared with Adult Rats." *Alcoholism: Clinical and Experimental Research* 24, no. 11 (Nov 2000): 1712–23.

Crews, Fulton T., A. Mdzinarishvili, D. Kim, J. He, and K. Nixon. "Neurogenesis in Adolescent Brains Is Potently Inhibited by Ethanol." *Neuroscience* 137 (2006): 437–45.

Crowley, Thomas J., and Paula D. Riggs. "Adolescent Substance Use Disorder with Conduct Disorder and Comorbid Conditions." In *National Institute on Drug Abuse Research Monograph No. 156*, edited by Elizabeth Rahdert and Dorynne Czechowicz, 49–111. Rockville, MD: National Institutes of Health, Public Health Service, U.S. Department of Health and Human Services, 1995.

Cushman, Paul, Jr. "Abstinence Following Detoxification and Methadone Maintenance Treatment." *American Journal of Medicine* 65, no. 1 (Jul 1978): 46–52.

Dani, John A., Thomas R. Kosten, and Neal L. Benowitz. "The Pharmacology of Nicotine and Tobacco." Chap. 12 in *Principles of Addiction Medicine*, edited by Richard K. Ries, D. A. Fiellin and Shannon C. Miller, 179–91. Philadelphia: Lippincott, Williams & Wilkins, 2009.

D'Aunno, T., and H. A. Pollack. "Changes in Methadone Treatment Practices: Results from a National Panel Study, 1988–2000." *JAMA* 288, no. 7 (Aug 21, 2002): 850–56.

Degenhardt, L., L. Dierker, W. T. Chiu, M. E. Medina-Mora, Y. Neumark, N. Sampson, J. Alonso, et al. "Evaluating the Drug Use "Gateway" Theory Using Cross-National Data: Consistency and Associations of the Order of Initiation of Drug Use among Participants in the WHO World Mental Health Surveys." *Drug and Alcohol Dependence* 108, no. 1–2 (Apr 1, 2010): 84–97.

Dole, Vincent P. "Narcotic Addiction, Physical Dependence and Relapse." *New England Journal of Medicine* 286, no. 18 (May 4, 1972): 988–92.

Dole, Vincent P., Marie E. Nyswander, and Mary Jeanne Kreek. "Narcotic Blockade." *Archives of Internal Medicine* 118, no. 4 (Oct 1966): 304–9.

D'Onofrio, Gail, David A. Fiellin, Michael V. Pantalon, Marek C. Chawarski, Patricia H. Owens, Linda C. Degutis, Susan H. Busch, Steven L. Bernstein, and Patrick G. O'Connor. "A Brief Intervention Reduces Hazardous and Harmful Drinking in Emergency Department Patients." *Annals of Emergency Medicine* 60, no. 2 (Aug 2012): 181–92.

Doremus, Tamara L., Steven C. Brunell, Pottayil Rajendran, and Linda P. Spear. "Factors Influencing Elevated Ethanol Consumption in Adolescent Relative to Adult Rats." *Alcoholism: Clinical and Experimental Research* 29, no. 10 (Oct 2005): 1796–808.

Drews, C. D., C. C. Murphy, M. Yeargin-Allsopp, and P. Decoufle. "The Relationship between Idiopathic Mental Retardation and Maternal Smoking during Pregnancy." *Pediatrics* 97, no. 4 (Apr 1996): 547–53.

Dylan, Bob. *Lyrics, 1962–2001.* New York: Simon & Schuster, 2004.

Edelman, E. Jennifer, An Dinh, Radu Radulescu, Bonnie Lurie, Gail D'Onofrio, Jeanette M. Tetrault, David A. Fiellin, and Lynn E. Fiellin. "Combining Rapid HIV Testing and a Brief Alcohol Intervention in Young Unhealthy Drinkers in the Emergency Department: A Pilot Study." *American Journal of Drug and Alcohol Abuse* 38, no. 6 (Nov 2012): 539–43.

Egan, Brent, Yumin Zhao, and Neal Axon. "U.S. Trends in Prevalence, Awareness, Treatment, and Control of Hypertension." *JAMA* 303, no. 20 (2010): 2043–50.

Englund, Michelle M., B. Egeland, E. M. Oliva, and W. A. Collins. "Childhood and Adolescent Predictors of Heavy Drinking and Alcohol Use Disorders in Early Adulthood: A Longitudinal Developmental Analysis." *Addiction* 103, suppl 1 (May 2008): 23–35.

Englund, Michelle M., Jessica Siebenbruner, Elizabeth M. Oliva, Byron Egeland, Chu-Ting Chung, and Jeffrey D. Long. "The Developmental Significance of Late Adolescent Substance Use for Early Adult Functioning." *Developmental Psychology* 49, no. 8 (Oct 1, 2012): 1554–64.

Enoch, Mary-Anne. "Genetic and Environmental Influences on the Development of Alcoholism: Resilience vs. Risk." *Annals of the New York Academy of Sciences* 1094 (Dec 2006): 193–201.

Everitt, B. J., and T. W. Robbins. "Neural Systems of Reinforcement for Drug Addiction: From Actions to Habits to Compulsion." *Nature Neuroscience* 8 (2005): 1481–89.

Falk, Gerhard. *Stigma: How We Treat Outsiders.* Amherst, NY: Prometheus Books, 2001.

Federal Student Aid, an office of the U.S. Department of Education. "Incarcerated Individuals and Eligibility for Federal Student Aid." Edited by Federal Student Aid. Accessed Jun 5, 2013, http://studentaid.ed.gov/sites/default/files/aid-info-for-incarcerated-individuals.pdf.

Fillmore, K. M. "Relationships between Specific Drinking Problems in Early Adulthood and Middle Age." *Journal of Studies on Alcohol* 36 (1975): 882–907.

Finn, R., and J. Clancy. "Alcoholism, Dilemma or Disease: A Recurring Problem for the Physician." *Comprehensive Psychiatry* 13, no. 2 (Mar 1972): 133–38.

Fisher, Joseph C., Robert L. Mason, Kim A. Keeley, and Joseph V. Fisher. "Physicians and Alcoholics: The Effect of Medical Training on Attitudes toward Alcoholics." *Journal of Studies on Alcohol and Drugs* 36, no. 7 (Jul 1975): 949–55.

Fleming, Michael F., Marlon P. Mundt, Michael T. French, Linda Baier Manwell, Ellyn A. Stauffacher, and Kristen Lawton Barry. "Benefit-Cost Analysis of Brief Physician Advice with Problem Drinkers in Primary Care Settings." *Medical Care* 38, no. 1 (2000): 7–18.

Ford, Betty. "Testimony before Join Together Policy Panel." In *Ending Discrimination against People with Alcohol and Drug Problems: Recommendations from a National Policy Panel,* edited by Join Together. Boston: Boston University School of Public Health, 2002.

Frary, Carol D., Rachel K. Johnson, and Min Qi Wang. "Food Sources and Intakes of Caffeine in the Diets of Persons in the United States." *Journal of the American Dietetic Association* 105, no. 1 (Jan 2005): 110–13.

Freire, Paulo. *Pedagogy of Hope.* New York: Continuum, 1994.

———. *Pedagogy of the Oppressed.* Translated by Myra Bergman Ramos. New York: Seabury Press, 1970 (1968).

Friedman, Jennifer, and Marixsa Alicea. *Surviving Heroin: Interviews with Women in Methadone Clinics.* Gainesville: University Press of Florida, 2001.

Garfein, Richard S., Elizabeth T. Golub, Alan E. Greenberg, Holly Hagan, Debra L. Hanson, Sharon M. Hudson, Farzana Kapadia, et al. "A Peer-Education Intervention to Reduce Injection Risk Behaviors for HIV and Hepatitis C Virus Infection in Young Injection Drug Users." *Aids* 21, no. 14 (2007): 1923–32.

Gladwell, Malcolm. *The Tipping Point: How Little Things Can Make a Big Difference.* Boston: Back Bay Books, 2002.

Glueck, Sheldon, and Eleanor Glueck. *Delinquents and Nondelinquents in Perspective.* Cambridge, MA: Harvard University Press, 1968.

Gogtay, Nitin, Jay N. Giedd, Leslie Lusk, Kiralee M. Hayashi, Deanna Greenstein, A. Catherine Vaituzis, Tom F. Nugent, et al. "Dynamic Mapping of Human Cortical Development during Childhood through Early Adulthood." *Proceedings of the National Academy of Sciences of the United States of America* 101, no. 21 (2004): 8174–79.

Goldstein, Rita Z., and Nora D. Volkow. "Drug Addiction and Its Underlying Neurobiological Basis: Neuroimaging Evidence for the Involvement of the Frontal Cortex." *American Journal of Psychiatry* 159, no. 10 (Oct 2002): 1642–52.

———. "Dysfunction of the Prefrontal Cortex in Addiction: Neuroimaging Findings and Clinical Implications." *Nature Reviews Neuroscience* 12, no. 11 (Nov 2011): 652–69.

Goodman, Jordan. *Tobacco in History: The Cultures of Dependence.* Paperback ed. London: Routledge, 1994.

Griswold, Patrick, MD, and Hillary Jacobs. *Waking Up: A Film about Opiate Addiction and Recovery.* Funded by the Bonney Family Foundation and the Society for the Arts in Healthcare (RWJ), 2006.

Haack, Mary R., and Hoover Adger, Jr., eds. "Strategic Plan for Interdisciplinary Faculty Development: Arming the Nation's Health Professional Workforce for a New Approach to Substance Use Disorders." *Substance Abuse* 23, no. 3 (Sep 2002): 1–345.

Hansson, Lars, Henrika Jormfeldt, Petra Svedberg, and Bengt Svensson. "Mental Health Professionals' Attitudes Towards People with Mental Illness: Do They Differ from Attitudes Held by People with Mental Illness?" *International Journal of Social Psychiatry* 59, no. 1 (Feb 2013): 48–54.

Harrison Narcotics Tax Act. Public Law 223. 63rd Congress, Dec 14, 1914.

Hasin, Deborah S., Frederick S. Stinson, Elizabeth Ogburn, and Bridget F. Grant. "Prevalence, Correlates, Disability, and Comorbidity of DSM-IV Alcohol Abuse and Dependence in the United States: Results from the National Epidemiologic Survey on Alcohol and Related Conditions." *Archives of General Psychiatry* 64, no. 7 (Jul 2007): 830–42.

Hauser, Stuart T., Joseph P. Allen, and Eve Golden. *Out of the Woods: Tales of Resilient Teens*. Cambridge, MA: Harvard University Press, 2006.

Heron, Melonie. "Deaths: Leading Causes 2009." Edited by National Center for Vital Statistics. Hyattsville, MD: National Center for Health Statistics, 2012.

Himmelstein, David U., Deborah Thorne, Elizabeth Warren, and Steffie Woolhandler. "Medical Bankruptcy in the United States, 2007: Results of a National Study." *American Journal of Medicine* 122, no. 8 (2009): 741–46.

Holliday, J. S. *Rush for Riches: Gold Fever and the Making of California*. San Francisco: University of California Press, 1999.

Houghton, Eleni, and Ann M. Roche, eds. *Learning about Drinking*. Edited by Marcus Grant. International Center for Alcohol Policies Series on Alcohol and Society. Philadelphia: Taylor & Francis, 2001.

Hughes, J. C., and C. C. Cook. "The Efficacy of Disulfiram: A Review of Outcome Studies." *Addiction* 92, no. 4 (Apr 1997): 381–95.

Hughes, Jason. *Learning to Smoke: Tobacco Use in the West*. Chicago: University of Chicago Press, 2003.

Hurd, Y. L. "Perspectives on Current Directions in the Neurobiology of Addiction Disorders Relevant to Genetic Risk Factors." *CNS Spectrums* 11, no. 11 (Nov 2006): 855–62.

Hyman, Steven E. "Addiction: A Disease of Learning and Memory." *American Journal of Psychiatry* 162, no. 8 (Aug 2005): 1414–22.

———. "The Neurobiology of Addiction: Implications for Voluntary Control of Behavior." *American Journal of Bioethics* 7, no. 1 (Jan 2007): 8–11.

Hyman, Steven E., Robert C. Malenka, and Eric J. Nestler. "Neural Mechanisms of Addiction: The Role of Reward-Related Learning and Memory." *Annual Review of Neuroscience* 29 (Jul 21, 2006): 565–98.

Iacono, William G., Stephen M. Malone, and Matt McGue. "Behavioral Disinhibition and the Development of Early-Onset Addiction: Common and Specific Influences." *Annual Review of Clinical Psychology* 4 (2008): 325–48.

"Impaired Driving: Get the Facts." Centers for Disease Control and Prevention. Accessed May 12, 2013. www.cdc.gov.

Isaacson, J. Harry, Michael Fleming, Mark Kraus, Ruth Kahn, and Marlon Mundt. "A National Survey of Training in Substance Use Disorders in Residency Programs." *Journal of Studies on Alcohol and Drugs* 61, no. 6 (Nov 2000): 912–15.

Jackson, Donald Dale. *Gold Dust: The California Gold Rush and the Forty-Niners.* London: George Allen & Unwin, 1980.

Jessor, R. "Problem-Behavior Theory, Psychosocial Development and Adolescent Problem Drinking." *British Journal of Addictions* 82 (1987): 331–42.

Johnson, B. A., N. Rosenthal, J. A. Capece, F. Wiegand, L. Mao, K. Beyers, A. McKay, et al. "Topiramate for Treating Alcohol Dependence: A Randomized Controlled Trial." *JAMA* 298, no. 14 (Oct 10, 2007): 1641–51.

Johnson, J. L., and M. Leff. "Children of Substance Abusers: Overview of Research Findings." *Pediatrics* 1035 part 2 (1999): 1085–99.

Johnston, L. D., P. M. O'Malley, J. G. Bachman, and J. E. Schulenberg. "Monitoring the Future National Results on Adolescent Drug Use: Overview of Key Findings, 2005." National Institutes of Health, 2006.

———. "Monitoring the Future National Results on Drug Use: 2012 Overview; Key Findings on Adolescent Drug Use." Ann Arbor, MI: Institute for Social Research, University of Michigan, 2013.

Join Together Policy Panel, Kurt L. Schmoke, Esq., chair. "Ending Discrimination against People with Alcohol and Drug Problems." Boston University School of Public Health, 2003.

Kalman, David, Sandra Baker Morissette, and Tony P. George. "Co-morbidity of Smoking in Patients with Psychiatric and Substance Use Disorders." *American Journal on Addictions* 14, no. 2 (Mar–Apr 2005): 106–23.

Kaskutas, Lee Ann. "Alcoholics Anonymous Effectiveness: Faith Meets Science." *Journal of Addictive Diseases* 28, no. 2 (2009): 145–57.

Kelley, Ann E., and Kent C. Berridge. "The Neuroscience of Natural Rewards: Relevance to Addictive Drugs." *Journal of Neuroscience* 22, no. 9 (May 1, 2002): 3306–11.

Kessler, David A. *A Question of Intent: A Great American Battle with a Deadly Industry.* Cambridge, MA: The Perseus Books Group, 2001.

Kessler, David A., Sharon L. Natanblut, Judith P. Wilkenfeld, Catherine C. Lorraine, Sharon Lindan Mayl, Ilisa B. G. Bernstein, and Larry Thompson. "Nicotine Addiction: A Pediatric Disease." *Journal of Pediatrics* 130, no. 4 (1997): 518–24.

Kessler, Ronald C. "The Epidemiology of Dual Diagnosis." *Biological Psychiatry* 56, no. 10 (Nov 15, 2004): 730–37.

Kiefer, Falk, Holger Jahn, Timo Tarnaske, Hauke Helwig, Peer Briken, Rudiger Holzbach, Philipp Kampf, et al. "Comparing and Combining Naltrexone and Acamprosate in Relapse Prevention of Alcoholism: A Double-Blind, Placebo-Controlled Study." *Archives of General Psychiatry* 60, no. 1 (Jan 2003): 92–99.

Kim, Theresa W., Richard Saitz, Debbie M. Cheng, Michael R. Winter, Julie Witas, and Jeffrey H. Samet. "Effect of Quality Chronic Disease Management for Alcohol and Drug Dependence on Addiction Outcomes." *Journal of Substance Abuse Treatment* 43, no. 4 (Dec 2012): 389–96.

Klausner, Samuel Z., and Edward F. Foulks. *Eskimo Capitalists: Oil, Politics, and Alcohol.* Totowa, NJ: Allenheld, Osmun & Co., 1982.

Knight, John R., S. K. Harris, L. Sherritt, S. Van Hook, N. Lawrence, T. Brooks, P. Carey, R. Kossack, and J. Kulig. "Prevalence of Positive Substance Abuse

Screen Results among Adolescent Primary Care Patients." *Archives of Pediatrics and Adolescent Medicine* 161, no. 11 (Nov 2007): 1035–41.

Knight, John R., Lydia A. Shrier, Terrill D. Bravender, Michelle Farrell, Joni Vander Bilt, and Howard J. Shaffer. "A New Brief Screen for Adolescent Substance Abuse." *Archives of Pediatrics & Adolescent Medicine* 153, no. 6 (Jun 1999): 591–96.

Koob, George F. "Negative Reinforcement in Drug Addiction: The Darkness Within." *Current Opinion in Neurobiology* 23, no. 4 (Apr 26, 2013): 559–63.

———. "The Neurobiology of Addiction: A Neuroadaptational View Relevant for Diagnosis." *Addiction* 101, suppl 1 (2006): 23–30.

Koob, George F., and Michel Le Moal. "Drug Abuse: Hedonic Homeostatic Dysregulation." *Science* 278, no. 5335 (Oct 3, 1997): 52–58.

———. "Plasticity of Reward Neurocircuitry and the 'Dark Side' of Drug Addiction." *Nature Neuroscience* 8, no. 11 (Nov 2005): 1442–4.

Koren, G., I. Nulman, A. E. Chudley, and C. Loocke. "Fetal Alcohol Spectrum Disorder." *CMAJ* 169, no. 11 (Nov 25, 2003): 1181–85.

Kranzler, Henry R., Domenic A. Ciraulo, and Jerome H. Jaffe. "Medications for Use in Alcohol Rehabilitation." Chap. 46 in *Principles of Addiction Medicine,* edited by Richard K. Ries, David A. Fiellin, Shannon C. Miller, and Richard Saitz, 631–43. Philadelphia: Lippincott, Williams & Wilkins, 2009.

Kranzler, Henry R., and Allyson Gage. "Acamprosate Efficacy in Alcohol-Dependent Patients: Summary of Results from Three Pivotal Trials." *American Journal on Addictions* 17, no. 1 (Jan–Feb 2008): 70–76.

Kranzler, Henry R., and Richard N. Rosenthal. "Dual Diagnosis: Alcoholism and Co-morbid Psychiatric Disorders." *American Journal on Addictions* 12, no. s1 (2003): S26–40.

Kreek, Mary Jeanne, David A. Nielsen, Eduardo R. Butelman, and Steven K. LaForge. "Genetic Influences on Impulsivity, Risk Taking, Stress Responsivity and Vulnerability to Drug Abuse and Addiction." *Nature Neuroscience* 8, no. 11 (2005): 1450–59.

Langdon, E. Jean Matteson. "Dau: Shamanic Power in Siona Religion." In *Portals of Power,* edited by E. Jean Matteson Langdon and Gerhard Baer. Albuquerque: University of New Mexico Press, 1992.

———. "Shamanism and Anthropology." In *Portals of Power: Shamanism in South America* edited by E. Jean Matteson Langdon and Gerhard Baer, 21. Albuquerque: University of New Mexico Press, 1992.

Langman, Louise, and Man Cheung Chung. "The Relationship between Forgiveness, Spirituality, Traumatic Guilt and Posttraumatic Stress Disorder (PTSD) among People with Addiction." *Psychiatric Quarterly* (2013): 1–16.

Lasser, Karen, J. Wesley Boyd, Stephanie Woolhandler, David Himmelstein, Daniel McCormick, and David Bor. "Smoking and Mental Illness: A Population-Based Prevalence Study." *JAMA* 284, no. 20 (2000): 2606–10.

Leis, Roberta, and David Rosenbloom. "The Road from Addiction Recovery to Productivity: Ending Discrimination against People with Alcohol and Drug Problems." *Family Court Review* 47 (2009): 274–85.

Lemanski, Michael. *A History of Addiction and Recovery in the United States.* Tucson, AZ: See Sharp Press, 2001.

Levin, E. D. "Persisting Effects of Chronic Adolescent Nicotine Administration on Radial-Arm Maze Learning and Response to Nicotine Challenges." *Neurotoxicology and Teratology* 21 (1999): 338.

Li, Ming D., and Margit Burmeister. "New Insights into the Genetics of Addiction." *Nature Reviews Genetics* 10 (2009): 225–31.

Little, Patrick J., Cynthia M. Kuhn, Wilkie A. Wilson, and H. Scott Swartzwelder. "Differential Effects of Ethanol in Adolescent and Adult Rats." *Alcoholism: Clinical and Experimental Research* 20, no. 8 (Nov 1996): 1346–51.

Logan, D. E., and G. A. Marlatt. "Harm Reduction Therapy: A Practice-Friendly Review of Research." *Journal of Clinical Psychology* 66, no. 2 (Feb 2010): 201–14.

Lorig, Kate R., and Halsted R. Holman. "Self-Management Education: History, Definition, Outcomes, and Mechanisms." *Annals of Behavioral Medicine* 26, no. 1 (Aug 2003): 1–7.

MacMullan, Jackie. *Boston Globe*, Jun 25, 1986.

Marcus, Marianne T. "Final Progress Report. HRSA-AMERSA-SAMHSA/CSAT Interdisciplinary Program to Improve Health Professional Education in Substance Abuse. Grant No.: 1u78 Hp 00001–03." Providence, RI: Association for Medical Education and Research in Substance Abuse (AMERSA), 2006.

Markwiese, Barbara J., Shawn K. Acheson, Edward D. Levin, Wilkie A. Wilson, and H. Scott Swartzwelder. "Differential Effects of Ethanol on Memory in Adolescent and Adult Rats." *Alcoholism: Clinical and Experimental Research* 22, no. 2 (Apr 1998): 416–21.

Masten, Ann S., and Anne Shaffer. "How Families Matter in Child Development: Reflections from Research on Risk and Resilience." In *Families Count: Effects of Child and Adolescent Development*, edited by Alison Clarke-Stewart and Judy Dunn, 5–25. New York: Cambridge University Press, 2006.

Matthew. "The Gospel According to Matthew." In *The New Testament of Our Lord and Savior Jesus Christ*. New York: The World Publishing Company, 1962.

McCord, W., and J. McCord. *Origins of Alcoholism*. Stanford, CA: Stanford University Press, 1960.

McGlynn, Elizabeth A., Steven M. Asch, John Adams, Joan Keesey, Jennifer Hicks, Alison DeCristofaro, and Eve A. Kerr. "The Quality of Health Care Delivered to Adults in the United States." *New England Journal of Medicine* 348, no. 26 (Jun 26, 2003): 2635–45.

McLellan, A. Thomas, and Kathleen Meyers. "Contemporary Addiction Treatment: A Review of Systems Problems for Adults and Adolescents." *Biological Psychiatry* 56, no. 10 (Nov 15, 2004): 764–70.

Meaney, Michael J. "Maternal Care, Gene Expression, and the Transmission of Individual Differences in Stress Reactivity across Generations." *Annual Review of Neuroscience* 24 (2001): 1161–92.

Merlin, Mark D. *On the Trail of the Ancient Opium Poppy*. Cranbury, NJ: Associated University Press, 1984.

Merrill, J. O., L. A. Rhodes, R. A. Deyo, G. A. Marlatt, and K. A. Bradley. "Mutual Mistrust in the Medical Care of Drug Users: The Keys to the "Narc" Cabinet." *Journal of General Internal Medicine* 17, no. 5 (May 2002): 327–33.

Miller, Brian T., and Mark D'Esposito. "Searching for 'the Top' in Top-Down Control." *Neuron* 48, no. 4 (2005): 535–38.

Miller, Norman S., Lorinda M. Sheppard, Christopher C. Colenda, and Jed Magen. "Why Physicians Are Unprepared to Treat Patients Who Have Alcohol- and Drug-Related Disorders." *Academic Medicine* 76, no. 5 (May 2001): 410–18.

Miller, T., and D. Hendrie. "Substance Abuse Prevention Dollars and Cents: A Cost-Benefit Analysis." Edited by Substance Abuse and Mental Health Services Administration Center for Substance Abuse Prevention. Rockville, MD: U.S. Department of Health and Human Services, 2008.

Miller, William R., R. Gayle Benefield, and J. Scott Tonigan. "Enhancing Motivation for Change in Problem Drinking: A Controlled Comparison of Two Therapist Styles." *Journal of Consulting and Clinical Psychology* 61 (1993): 455–61.

Miller, William R., and Stephen Rollnick. *Motivational Interviewing: Preparing People for Change.* 2nd ed. New York: Guilford Press, 2002.

Miller, William R., Scott T. Walters, and Melanie E. Bennett. "How Effective Is Alcoholism Treatment in the United States?" *Journal of Studies on Alcohol and Drugs* 62, no. 2 (Mar 2001): 211–20.

Miner, Lucinda. "Neurobiology of Addiction." In *Clinical Teaching in Addiction Medicine: A Chief Resident Immersion Training (CRIT) Program.* Chatham, MA, 2006.

Miniño, A. M., and S. L. Murphy. "Death in the United States, 2010." Hyattsville, MD, 2012.

Monti, Peter M., Robert Miranda, Kimberly Nixon, Kenneth J. Sher, H. Scott Swartzwelder, Susan F. Tapert, Aaron White, and Fulton T. Crews. "Adolescence: Booze, Brains, and Behavior." *Alcoholism: Clinical and Experimental Research* 29, no. 2 (Feb 2005): 207–20.

Moos, Rudolf H., and Bernice S. Moos. "Participation in Treatment and Alcoholics Anonymous: A 16-Year Follow-up of Initially Untreated Individuals." *Journal of Clinical Psychology* 62, no. 6 (Jun 2006): 735–50.

Musto, David F. *The American Disease: Origins of Narcotic Control.* 3rd ed. New York: Oxford University Press, 1999.

National Institute on Alcohol Abuse and Alcoholism. "A Clinician's Guide to Alcohol Use." National Institutes of Health, 2004.

———. "Helping Patients Who Drink Too Much: A Clinician's Guide." National Institutes of Health, 2005.

National Institutes of Health. "The NIH Almanac." NIH. Accessed Jun 2, 2013. www.nih.gov.

Nixon, Kimberly, and Fulton T. Crews. "Binge Ethanol Exposure Decreases Neurogenesis in Adult Rat Hippocampus." *Journal of Neurochemistry* 83, no. 5 (Dec 2002): 1087–93.

Noaj, Benei, ed. *Alcoholics Anonymous Big Book: Special Edition Including New Personal Stories for the Year 2007.* AA Services, 2006.

Obernier, Jennifer A., T. W. Bouldin, and F. T. Crews. "Binge Ethanol Exposure in Adult Rats Causes Necrotic Cell Death." *Alcoholism: Clinical and Experimental Research* 26, no. 4 (Apr 2002): 547–57.

Obernier, Jennifer A., Aaron M. White, H. Scott Swartzwelder, and Fulton T. Crews. "Cognitive Deficits and CNS Damage after a 4-Day Binge Ethanol Exposure in Rats." *Pharmacology Biochemistry and Behavior* 72, no. 3 (Jun 2002): 521–32.

Patient Protection and Affordable Care Act of 2010. Public Law 111-148, 124 Stat. 119 (2010).

Peabody, Francis Weld. *Doctor and Patient.* New York: MacMillan Company, 1930.

Personal Responsibility and Work Opportunity Reconciliation Act. Public. Law. no. 104-193, Sect. 115, 110 Stat. 2105 (1996).

Pistis, Marco, Simona Perra, Giuliano Pillolla, Miriam Melis, Anna Lisa Muntoni, and Gian Luigi Gessa. "Adolescent Exposure to Cannabinoids Induces Long-Lasting Changes in the Response to Drugs of Abuse of Rat Midbrain Dopamine Neurons." *Biological psychiatry* 56, no. 2 (Jul 15, 2004): 86–94.

Pollan, Michael. *The Botany of Desire.* New York: Random House, 2001.

Prendergast, Michael L., Deborah Podus, Eunice Chang, and Darren Urada. "The Effectiveness of Drug Abuse Treatment: A Meta-analysis of Comparison Group Studies." *Drug and Alcohol Dependence* 67 (2002): 53–72.

Prochaska, James O., and Carlo C. DiClemente. "Stages and Process of Self Change in Smoking: Toward an Integrative Model of Change." *Journal of Consulting and Clinical Psychology* 51 (1983): 390–97.

Pyapali, G. K., D. A. Turner, W. A. Wilson, and H. S. Swartzwelder. "Age and Dose-Dependent Effects of Ethanol on the Induction of Hippocampal Long-Term Potentiation." *Alcohol* 19 no. 2 (Oct 1999): 107–11.

The Qur'an: A Modern English Version. Translated by Majid Fakhry. Paperback ed. Reading, UK: Garnet Publishing, 1997. doi:http://www.studytoanswer.net /islam/badwine.html.

Rasyidi, Ernest, Jeffery N. Wilkins, and Itai Danovitch. "Training the Next Generation of Providers in Addiction Medicine." *Psychiatric Clinics of North America* 35, no. 2 (Jun 2012): 461–80.

Rettig, Richard A., and Adam Yarmolinsky, eds. *Federal Regulation of Methadone Treatment Institute of Medicine.* Washington, DC: National Academies Press, 1995.

Rigotti, N. A. "Strategies to Help a Smoker Who Is Struggling to Quit." *JAMA* 308, no. 15 (Oct 17, 2012): 1573–80.

Robbins, T. W., and B. J. Everitt. "Drug Addiction: Bad Habits Add Up." *Nature* 398, no. 6728 (Apr 15, 1999): 567–70.

Robins, Lee. *Deviant Children Grown Up.* Baltimore: The Williams and Wilkins Company, 1966.

Robinson, T. E., and K. C. Berridge. "Addiction." *Annual Review of Psychology* 54 (2003): 25–53.

Rohman, M. E., P. D. Cleary, M. Warburg, T. L. Delbanco, and M. D. Aronson. "The Response of Primary Care Physicians to Problem Drinkers." *American Journal of Drug and Alcohol Abuse* 13, no. 1–2 (1987): 199–209.

Room, Robin. "Stigma, Social Inequality and Alcohol and Drug Use." *Drug and Alcohol Review* 24, no. 2 (Mar 2005): 143–55.

Roosevelt, Franklin Delano. "Second Inaugural Address." Washington, DC, 1937.

Rorabaugh, W. J. *The Alcoholic Republic: An American Tradition.* New York: Oxford University Press, 1979.

Rosen, Tove S., and Helen L. Johnson. "Long-Term Effects of Prenatal Methadone Maintenance." National Institute on Drug Abuse (NIDA) Monograph 59 (1985): 73–83.

Rumbarger, John J. *Profits, Power, and Prohibition: Alcohol Reform and the Industrializing of America, 1800–1930.* SUNY Series in New Social Studies on Alcohol and Drugs. Albany: State University of New York Press, 1989.

Rush, Benjamin. *An Inquiry into the Effects of Ardent Spirits upon the Human Body and Mind.* 6th ed. New York: Lorig, 1811.

Rutherford, Helena J. V., Linda C. Mayes, and Marc N. Potenza. "Neurobiology of Adolescent Substance Use Disorders: Implications for Prevention and Treatment." *Child and Adolescent Psychiatric Clinics of North America* 19, no. 3 (Jul 2010): 479–92.

Rutter, Michael. "Developmental Catch-up, and Deficit, Following Adoption after Severe Global Early Privation." *Journal of Child Psychology and Psychiatry* 39, no. 4 (May 1998): 465–76.

———. *Genes and Behavior: Nature-Nurture Interplay Explained.* Oxford, UK: Blackwell Publishing, 2006.

———. "Implications of Resilience Concepts for Scientific Understanding." *Annals of the New York Academy of Sciences* 1094 (2006): 1–12.

———. "The Promotion of Resilience in the Face of Adversity." In *Families Count: Effects on Child and Adolescent Development,* edited by Alison Clarke-Stewart and Judy Dunn, 26–52. New York: Cambridge University Press, 2006.

Saitz, Richard, Mary Jo Larson, Colleen LaBelle, Jessica Richardson, and Jeffrey H. Samet. "The Case for Chronic Disease Management for Addiction." *Journal of Addiction Medicine* 2, no. 2 (2008): 55.

Sameroff, Arnold J., and Katherine L. Rosenblum. "Psychosocial Constraints on the Development of Resilience." *Annals of the New York Academy of Sciences* 1094 (Dec 2006): 116–24.

Samet, Jeffrey H., and Patrick G. O'Connor. "Alcohol Abusers in Primary Care: Readiness to Change Behavior." *American Journal of Medicine* 105, no. 4 (1998): 302–6.

Saxon, Andrew J., Michael R. Oreskovich, and Zoran Brkanac. "Genetic Determinants of Addiction to Opioids and Cocaine." *Harvard Review of Psychiatry* 13, no. 4 (Jul–Aug 2005): 218–32.

Schippers, Gerard M., Marcel A. G. van Aken, Sylvia M. M. Lammers, and Laura de Fuentes Merillas. "Acquiring the Competence to Drink Responsibly." In *Learning About Drinking,* edited by Eleni Houghton and Ann M. Roche. International Center for Alcohol Policies Series on Alcohol and Society, 304. Philadelphia: Taylor & Francis, 2001.

Schlink, Bernhard. *The Reader.* Translated by Carol Brown Janeway. New York: Pantheon Books, 1997.

Schultz, Wolfram. "Behavioral Theories and the Neurophysiology of Reward." *Annual Review of Psychology* 57 (2006): 87–115.

Schweinsburg, Alecia D., Bonnie J. Nagel, and Susan F. Tapert. "FMRI Reveals Alteration of Spatial Working Memory Networks across Adolescence." *Journal of the International Neuropsychological Society* 11, no. 5 (Sep 2005): 631–44.

Scragg, Robert, Murray Laugesen, and Elizabeth Robinson. "Parental Smoking and Related Behaviours Influence Adolescent Tobacco Smoking: Results from the 2001 New Zealand National Survey of 4th Form Students." *New Zealand Medical Journal* 116, no. 1187 (Dec 12, 2003): U707.

Seeman, Teresa E., George A. Kaplan, Lisa Knudsen, Richard Cohen, and Jack Guralnik. "Social Network Ties and Mortality among the Elderly in the Alameda County Study." *American Journal of Epidemiology* 126, no. 4 (Oct 1987): 714–23.

Shakespeare, William. *The Tragedy of Hamlet.* The Kittredge Shakespeare. Edited by George L Kittredge. Boston: Ginn, 1939.

Shedler, Jonathan, and Jack Block. "Adolescent Drug Use and Psychological Health: A Longitudinal Inquiry." *American Psychologist* 45, no. 5 (May 1990): 612–30.

Sher, Kenneth J., Beth S. Gershuny, Lizette Peterson, and Gail Raskin. "The Role of Childhood Stressors in the Intergenerational Transmission of Alcohol Use Disorders." *Journal of Studies on Alcohol and Drugs* 58, no. 4 (1997): 414–27.

Siciliano, Denise, and Robert F. Smith. "Periadolescent Alcohol Alters Adult Behavioral Characteristics in the Rat." *Physiology and Behavior* 74 (2001): 637–43.

Siebenbruner, J., M. M. Englund, B. Egeland, and K. Hudson. "Developmental Antecedents of Late Adolescence Substance Use Patterns." *Development and Psychopathology* 18, no. 2 (Spring 2006): 551–71.

Skeem, Jennifer L., John Encandela, and Jennifer Eno Louden. "Perspectives on Probation and Mandated Mental Health Treatment in Specialized and Traditional Probation Departments." *Behavioral Sciences and the Law* 21 (2003): 429–58.

Skinner, Natalie, N. T. Feather, Toby Freeman, and Ann Roche. "Stigma and Discrimination in Health-Care Provision to Drug Users: The Role of Values, Affect, and Deservingness Judgments." *Journal of Applied Social Psychology* 37, no. 1 (2007): 163–86.

Slawecki, Craig J., Michelle Betancourt, Maury Cole, and Cindy L. Ehlers. "Periadolescent Alcohol Exposure Has Lasting Effects on Adult Neurophysiological Function in Rats." *Developmental Brain Research* 128, no. 1 (May 31, 2001): 63–72.

Slotkin, Theodore A., and Frederic J. Seidler. "Nicotine Exposure in Adolescence Alters the Response of Serotonin Systems to Nicotine Administered Subsequently in Adulthood." *Developmental Neuroscience* 31, no. 1–2 (2009): 58–70.

Smith, Robert F. "Animal Models of Periadolescent Substance Abuse." *Neurotoxicology and Teratology* 25, no. 3 (2003): 291–301.

Smith, Robert F., C. N. Medici, and D. K. Raap. "Enduring Behavioral Effects of Weaning-through-Puberty Cocaine Dosing in the Rat." *Psychobiology* 27 (1999): 432–37.

Solberg, Leif I., Michael V. Maciosek, and Nichol M. Edwards. "Primary Care Intervention to Reduce Alcohol Misuse: Ranking Its Health Impact and Cost Effectiveness." *American Journal of Preventive Medicine* 34, no. 2 (2008): 143–52.

Somerville, Leah H., and B. J. Casey. "Developmental Neurobiology of Cognitive Control and Motivational Systems." *Current Opinion in Neurobiology* 20, no. 2 (Apr 2010): 236–41.

Sowell, Elizabeth R., Paul M. Thompson, Kevin D. Tessner, and Arthur W. Toga. "Mapping Continued Brain Growth and Gray Matter Density Reduction in

Dorsal Frontal Cortex: Inverse Relationships during Postadolescent Brain Maturation." *Journal of Neuroscience* 21, no. 22 (Nov 15, 2001): 8819–29.

Sowell, Elizabeth R., Paul M. Thompson, and Arthur W. Toga. "Mapping Changes in the Human Cortex throughout the Span of Life." *Neuroscientist* 10, no. 4 (Aug 2004): 372–92.

Spear, Linda. "The Teenage Brain: Adolescents and Alcohol." *Current Directions in Psychological Science* 22, no. 2 (2013): 152–57.

Srisurapanont, Manit, and Ngamwong Jarusuraisin. "Naltrexone for the Treatment of Alcoholism: A Meta-analysis of Randomized Controlled Trials." *International Journal of Neuropsychopharmacology* 8, no. 2 (Jun 2005): 267–80.

Sroufe, L. Alan, Byron Egeland, Elizabeth A. Carlson, and W. Andrew Collins. *The Development of the Person: The Minnesota Study of Risk and Adaptation from Birth to Adulthood.* New York: Guilford Press, 2005.

Stehman, Christine R., and Mark B. Mycyk. "A Rational Approach to the Treatment of Alcohol Withdrawal in the ED." *American Journal of Emergency Medicine* 31, no. 4 (Apr 2013): 734–42.

Stewart, Jane. "Stress and Relapse to Drug Seeking: Studies in Laboratory Animals Shed Light on Mechanisms and Sources of Long-Term Vulnerability." *American Journal on Addictions* 12, no. 1 (Jan–Feb 2003): 1–17.

Stewart, William. *The Surgeon General's Report on Smoking: 1968 Supplement to Public Health Service Publication 1696.* Edited by U.S. Department of Health. U.S. Printing Office, 1968.

Stimmel, Barry, J. Goldberg, E. Rothopf, and M. Cohen. "Ability to Remain Abstinent after Methadone Detoxification: A Six-Year Study." *JAMA* 237, no. 12 (Mar 21, 1977): 1216–20.

Stine, Susan M., and Thomas R. Kosten. "Pharmacologic Interventions for Opioid Dependence." Chap. 48 in *Principles of Addiction Medicine, Fourth Edition,* edited by Richard K. Ries, David A. Fiellin, Shannon C. Miller, and Richard Saitz. Philadelphia: Lippincott, Williams, & Wilkins, 2009.

Strong, Moriah N., Naomi Yoneyama, Andrea M. Fretwell, Chris Snelling, Michelle A. Tanchuck, and Deborah A. Finn. "'Binge' Drinking Experience in Adolescent Mice Shows Sex Differences and Elevated Ethanol Intake in Adulthood." *Hormones and Behavior* 58, no. 1 (2010): 82–90.

Sturm, Roland, Weiying Zhang, and Michael Schoenbaum. "How Expensive Are Unlimited Substance Abuse Benefits under Managed Care?" *Journal of Behavioral Health Services & Research* 26, no. 2 (1999): 203–10.

Substance Abuse and Mental Health Services Administration. "National Household Survey on Drug Abuse." Ed. Applied Services Office, 1998.

———. "Results from the 2011 National Survey on Drug Use and Health: Summary of National Findings," 52, 89–98. Rockville, MD: Substance Abuse and Mental Health Services Administration, 2012.

Swartzwelder, H. S., R. C. Richardson, B. Markwiese-Foerch, W. A. Wilson, and P. J. Little. "Developmental Differences in the Acquisition of Tolerance to Ethanol." *Alcohol* 15, no. 4 (May 1998): 311–314.

Tomaka, Joe, Sharon Thompson, and Rebecca Palacios. "The Relation of Social

Isolation, Loneliness, and Social Support to Disease Outcomes among the Elderly." *Journal of Aging and Health* 18, no. 3 (Jun 2006): 359–84.

Torgoff, Martin. *Can't Find My Way Home.* New York: Simon & Schuster, 2004.

Trauth, Jennifer A., F. J. Seidler, E. C. McCook, and T. A. Slotkin. "Adolescent Nicotine Exposure Causes Persistent Upregulation of Nicotinic Cholinergic Receptors in Rat Brain Regions." *Brain Research* 851, no. 1–2 (Dec 18, 1999): 9–19.

Trauth, Jennifer A., Frederic J. Seidler, Syed F. Ali, and Theodore A. Slotkin. "Adolescent Nicotine Exposure Produces Immediate and Long-Term Changes in CNS Noradrenergic and Dopaminergic Function." *Brain Research* 892, no. 2 (Feb 23, 2001): 269–80.

Tronson, Natalie C., and Jane R. Taylor. "Addiction: A Drug-Induced Disorder of Memory Reconsolidation." *Current Opinion in Neurobiology* 23, no. 4 (Aug 2013): 573–80.

Tsoh, Janice Y., Felicia W. Chi, Jennifer R. Mertens, and Constance M. Weisner. "Stopping Smoking during First Year of Substance Use Treatment Predicted 9-Year Alcohol and Drug Treatment Outcomes." *Drug and Alcohol Dependence* 114, no. 2 (2011): 110–18.

U.S. Bureau of Labor Statistics. Accessed Mar 22, 2006. www.bls.gov.

U.S. Department of Health and Human Services. "Healthy People 2020: Topics and Objectives." Accessed Jun 5, 2013. www.healthypeople.gov.

U.S. Department of Labor. "Fact Sheet: The Mental Health Parity and Addiction Equity Act of 2008 (MHPAEA)." Accessed Jun 5, 2013. www.dol.gov.

U.S. Food and Drug Administration. "Nicotine Replacement Therapy Labels May Change." Department of Health and Human Services. Accessed Jul 21, 2013. www.fda.gov.

U.S. Institute of Medicine. *Broadening the Base of Treatment for Alcohol Problems.* Washington, DC: National Academies Press, 1990.

———, Committee on Crossing the Quality Chasm: Adaptation to Mental Health and Addictive Disorders. *Improving the Quality of Health Care for Mental and Substance-Use Conditions.* Quality Chasm Series. Edited by Institute of Medicine. Washington, DC: National Academies Press, 2006.

U.S. v. Doremus, 86 U.S. 249 (1919).

Vaillant, George E. *The Natural History of Alcoholism: Causes, Patterns, and Paths to Recovery.* Cambridge, MA: Harvard University Press, 1983.

———. *The Natural History of Alcoholism Revisited.* Cambridge, MA: Harvard University Press, 1995; repr., 2000.

———. *Triumphs of Experience: The Men of the Harvard Grant Study.* Cambridge, MA: The Belknap Press of Harvard University Press, 2012.

Varlinskaya, Elena I., and Linda P. Spear. "Acute Ethanol Withdrawal (Hangover) and Social Behavior in Adolescent and Adult Male and Female Sprague-Dawley Rats." *Alcoholism: Clinical and Experimental Research* 28, no. 1 (Jan 2004): 40–50.

———. "Differences in the Social Consequences of Ethanol Emerge during the Course of Adolescence in Rats: Social Facilitation, Social Inhibition, and Anxiolysis." *Developmental Psychobiology* 48, no. 2 (Mar 2006): 146–61.

Vega, William A., Sergio Aguilar-Gaxiola, Laura Andrade, Rob Bijl, Guilherme

Borges, Jorge J. Caraveo-Anduaga, David J. DeWit, et al. "Prevalence and Age of Onset for Drug Use in Seven International Sites: Results from the International Consortium of Psychiatric Epidemiology." *Drug and Alcohol Dependence* 68, no. 3 (2002): 285–97.

"Vital Signs: Overdoses of Prescription Opioid Pain Relievers—United States, 1998–2008." *Morbidity and Mortality Weekly Report* 60, no. 43 (2011): 1487–92. Accessed May 12, 2013. www.cdc.gov.

Volkow, N. D., Joanna S. Fowler, and Gene-Jack Wang. "The Addicted Human Brain Viewed in the Light of Imaging Studies: Brain Circuits and Treatment Strategies." *Neuropharmacology* 47, suppl 1 (2004): 3–13.

Volkow, Nora D., and Joanna S. Fowler. "Addiction, a Disease of Compulsion and Drive: Involvement of the Orbitofrontal Cortex." *Cerebral Cortex* 10 (2000): 318–25.

Volkow, Nora D., Gene-Jack Wang, Joanna S. Fowler, and Dardo Tomasi. "Addiction Circuitry in the Human Brain." *Annual Review of Pharmacology and Toxicology* 52 (2012): 321–36.

Volkow, Nora D., Gene-Jack Wang, Dardo Tomasi, and Ruben D. Baler. "Unbalanced Neuronal Circuits in Addiction." *Current Opinion in Neurobiology* 23, no. 4 (Aug 2013): 639–48.

Warren, Kenneth R., Brenda G. Hewitt, and Jennifer D. Thomas. "Fetal Alcohol Spectrum Disorders: Research Challenges and Opportunities." *Alcohol Research & Health* 34, no. 1 (2011).

Webb v. U.S., 249 U.S. 96 (1919).

Weber, Ellen M. "Equality Standards for Health Insurance Coverage: Will the Mental Health Parity and Addiction Equity Act End the Discrimination" (2012). *Golden Gate University Law Review* 43, no. 2 (2013).

Wegner, Daniel M. *The Illusion of Conscious Will*. Cambridge, MA: The MIT Press, 2002.

Weisner, Constance, Helen Matzger, Tammy Tam, and Laura Schmidt. "Who Goes to Alcohol and Drug Treatment? Understanding Utilization within the Context of Insurance." *Journal of Studies on Alcohol and Drugs* 63 (2002): 673–82.

Weisner, Constance, G. Thomas Ray, Jennifer R. Mertens, Derek D. Satre, and Charles Moore. "Short-Term Alcohol and Drug Treatment Outcomes Predict Long-Term Outcome." *Drug and Alcohol Dependence* 71, no. 3 (Sep 10, 2003): 281–94.

West, S. L., and K. K. O'Neal. "Project D.A.R.E. Outcome Effectiveness Revisited." *American Journal of Public Health* 94, no. 6 (2004).

Westermeyer, Joe, Linda Bennett, Paul Thuras, and Gihyun Yoon. "Substance Use Disorder among Adoptees: A Clinical Comparative Study." *American Journal of Drug and Alcohol Abuse* 33, no. 3 (2007): 455–66.

White, Aaron M., Amol J. Ghia, Edward D. Levin, and H. Scott Swartzwelder. "Binge Pattern Ethanol Exposure in Adolescent and Adult Rats: Differential Impact on Subsequent Responsiveness to Ethanol." *Alcoholism: Clinical and Experimental Research* 24, no. 8 (Aug 2000): 1251–56.

White, Aaron M., and H. Scott Swartzwelder. "Age-Related Effects of Alcohol on Memory and Memory-Related Brain Function in Adolescents and Adults." *Recent Developments in Alcoholism* 17 (2005): 161–76.

White, Aaron M., Melanie C. Truesdale, Jon G. Bae, Sukaina Ahmad, Wilkie A. Wilson, Phillip J. Best, and H. Scott Swartzwelder. "Differential Effects of Ethanol on Motor Coordination in Adolescent and Adult Rats." *Pharmacology Biochemistry and Behavior* 73, no. 3 (Oct 2002): 673–77.

WHO Brief Intervention Study Group. "A Randomized Cross-National Clinical Trial of Brief Intervention with Heavy Drinkers." *American Journal of Public Health* 86, no. 7 (1996): 948–55.

Wild, T. Cameron, Amanda B. Roberts, and Erin L. Cooper. "Compulsory Substance Abuse Treatment: An Overview of Recent Findings and Issues." *European Addiction Research* 8, no. 2 (2002): 84–93.

Wild, T. Cameron, Jody Wolfe, and Elaine Hyshka. "Consent and Coercion in Addiction Treatment." *Addiction Neuroethics: The Ethics of Addiction Neuroscience Research and Treatment* (2012): 153–74.

Williams, Geoffrey, Heather Patrick, Christopher Niemiec, L. Keoki Williams, George Devine, Jennifer Elston Lafata, Michele Heisler, Kaan Tunceli, and Manel Pladeval. "Reducing the Health Risks of Diabetes: How Self-Determination Theory May Help Improve Medication Theory and Quality of Life." *Diabetes Educator* 35, no. 3 (2009): 484–92.

Williams, William Carlos. *The Autobiography of William Carlos Williams.* New York: New Directions Books, 1951.

Wilson, G. B., C. A. Lock, N. Heather, P. Cassidy, M. M. Christie, and E. F. Kaner. "Intervention against Excessive Alcohol Consumption in Primary Health Care: A Survey of GPs' Attitudes and Practices in England 10 Years On." *Alcohol and Alcoholism* 46, no. 5 (Sep–Oct 2011): 570–77.

Wodak, Alex, and Annie Cooney. "Do Needle Syringe Programs Reduce HIV Infection among Injecting Drug Users: A Comprehensive Review of the International Evidence." *Substance Use & Misuse* 41, no. 6–7 (2006): 777–813.

Wordsworth, William. "My Heart Leaps up (1807)." In *The Norton Anthology of English Literature,* edited by M. H. Abrams, 1694. New York: W. W. Norton & Company, 1962.

World Health Organization. "The Tenth Revision of the International Classification of Diseases and Health Problems (ICD-9)." Accessed Jun 5, 2006. www.who.int.

Zailckas, Koren. *Smashed: Story of a Drunken Girlhood.* Paperback ed. New York: Penguin Group, 2006.

Zavala, A. R., A. Nazarian, C. A. Crawford, and S. A. McDougall. "Cocaine-Induced Behavioral Sensitization in the Young Rat." *Psychopharmacology (Berl)* 151, no. 2–3 (Aug 2000): 291–98.

INDEX

Page numbers in *italics* indicate figures and tables.

alcohol use (*continued*)
antidotes for overdoses of, 144; atypical, 62; binge drinking, 29, 31–32, 38, 64–65; and compulsive behavior, 44; family attitudes toward, 25; health risks of, 38; low risk and risky, 36–39; national guidelines, 36–39; normal, perceptions of, 37; numbing function of, 22; parental influences, 34–35; pharmacology of, 53, 56; progressive, 62; replacement therapy, 148–49, 151–52; social and economic costs of, 9–10; statistics on, 36–37; and stigma, 69–72, 75–76, 80–84, 87–88; and stress, 104; Study of Adult Development, 62–65; treatment by primary care providers, 137–38, *138*; as underlying cause of death, 10; universality of, 20; withdrawal from, 145–47; Zailckas on, 19, 22
alcohol use disorders (AUDs), 30, 35, 65, 128, 133, *139*
alleles, 103
Allen, Joseph P., 113
alprazolam (Xanax), 22, 105
American Society of Addiction Medicine, 86–87
amphetamines, 39, 52–53, 105, 144, 157
amygdala, 46, 49, 51–52, 60
anandamide, 53–54
animal studies on drug use, 29–32, 45–46, *46*, 49–52, 57–58, 96, 100, 102
Antabuse (disulfiram), 148–49
antagonist medication, 148
anterior cingulate cortex, 55, 105
anticipation, 11–12, 47, 51, 57, 59
antidepressants, 146, 152
antireward system, 56–57
anti-Semitism, 67–68
Association for Medical Education and Research in Substance Abuse (AMERSA), 85
Ativan, 147
atropine, 21

attention deficit hyperactivity disorder (ADHD), 104
AUDs. *See* alcohol use disorders
aversive conditioning, 148

Balint, Michael, 158
bankruptcy, 88
barbiturates, 22
Beck, Deb, 88, 89–90
behavior, changing, 127–30, *129*
Belladonna, 21
benzodiazepines, 22, 105, 142–43, 146, 151
beta-endorphins, 105
Betty Ford Center, 84
binge drinking, 29, 31–32, 38, 57, 64–65
Botany of Desire (Pollan), 20–21
Braceland, Tom, 64
brain development: adolescent response to drug use, 32–36; adolescent vs. adult response to drug use, 28–32; and individuation, 33; normal child and adolescent, 26–28, *28*; and plasticity, 26, 33, 55, 57
brain dysfunction, 5, 59–60
Brazil, Russell, 1–2, 15–17, 156
brief interventions, 137, 140
Broadening the Base of Treatment for Alcohol Problems, 84
buprenorphine, 51, 147, 149–52. *See also* Suboxone
bupropion, 152
Bureau of Health Professions, Health Resources and Services Administration (HRSA), 85
Burroughs, William, 23

caffeine, 11–12, 16, 23–25, 42–43
Cahalan, Dennis, 63
cannabinoids, 29, 32, 103. *See also* marijuana
caring relationships, 113, 115
case studies: Bill, 17, 47–48, 51, 73, 101–2, 111, 118, 123, 126, 132, 134, 140, 142, 155–56, 159; CF, 134; DC, 13–14; Delia, 17, 24, 55, 104, 118,